The Paris System for Reporting Urinary Cytology

Dorothy L. Rosenthal • Eva M. Wojcik
Daniel F.I. Kurtycz
Editors

The Paris System for Reporting Urinary Cytology

Springer

THE INTERNATIONAL ACADEMY OF CYTOLOGY
1957

ASC
AMERICAN SOCIETY OF Cytopathology
Saving Lives One Cell at a Time™

Editors
Dorothy L. Rosenthal
The Johns Hopkins Hospital
The Johns Hopkins University
Baltimore, MD, USA

Eva M. Wojcik
Department of Pathology
Loyola University Medical Center
Maywood, IL, USA

Daniel F.I. Kurtycz
Department of Pathology
and Laboratory Medicine
University of Wisconsin School of
Medicine and Public Health
Wisconsin State Laboratory of Hygiene
Madison, WI, USA

ISBN 978-3-319-22863-1 ISBN 978-3-319-22864-8 (eBook)
DOI 10.1007/978-3-319-22864-8

Library of Congress Control Number: 2015957589

Springer Cham Heidelberg New York Dordrecht London

Printed on acid-free paper

Springer International Publishing AG Switzerland is part of Springer Science+Business Media (www.springer.com)

To my husband, Bill, who taught me what it's like to live with bladder cancer.—DLR

To the men of my life—my husband, Mike, and my sons, Adam and Mark.—EMW

To my wife, Tina, who taught me how to dance.—DFK

Foreword

From Bethesda to Paris—At Last We Have Standardized Terminology for Urinary Cytology!

In our capacity as pathologists, we serve as consultants to our clinical colleagues and patients. Particularly in anatomic pathology, our reports are the documentation of this communication and constitute a major component of the patient's electronic medical record. To enable clinicians to choose the optimal management option(s) for their patient, it is imperative that these reports accurately, clearly, and predictably communicate our pathology findings. In anatomic pathology, especially in cytopathology, we variably use terms such as "suspicious," "indeterminate," or "atypical" to describe the same findings. The use of these equivocal terms varies among different pathologists and institutions leading to confusion among clinicians as well as patients, who in the present days, often have access to their reports. Both clinicians and pathologists have recognized the need for a more standardized terminology for reporting cytopathology results and for the education of the clinicians on that terminology. This issue is certainly not unique to cytopathology reports: in surgical pathology in spite of attempts to pay attention to completeness of reports (tumor staging summaries, etc.), up to 30 % of reports may be misunderstood by clinicians, in large part due to the variability of the wording by pathologists.

The Bethesda System (TBS) cervical cytology terminology effort, initiated in 1988, led the way for standardized reporting in cytopathology. TBS addressed specimen adequacy, correlated morphology with the biology of disease processes, "lumped" biologically equivalent entities, and recognized the necessity to improve interobserver reproducibility of the equivocal category of "atypia" based upon histopathology and clinical outcomes. After initial reluctance by the international community, TBS has achieved widespread international acceptance, leading to standardized terminology, corresponding management guidelines, and to funding of research. The Bethesda System has been the model for subsequent development of standardized cytopathology reporting consensus efforts in thyroid and pancreatic cytopathology, and for histopathology reporting of HPV-related lower genital tract terminology. In keeping with its goals and in recognition of its practical relevance, the cervical cytology Bethesda System has been updated over the years; the most recent update was finalized in 2014. In the area of non-gynecologic cytology reporting, the College of American Pathologists described major elements of quality non-gynecologic cytology reporting and encouraged the use of standardization of non-gynecologic terminology.

Urine cytology comprises a variable but significant percentage of daily non-gynecologic case volume in many cytopathology practices. Despite two well-established pathways and risk-based prognostic categories for urothelial carcinoma, the cytologic terminology for urinary cytology remains disparate and complex. Similar terminology problems existed for Pap tests prior to Bethesda 1988 and for thyroid FNA prior to Bethesda 2007. In 2004, the Papanicolaou Society of Cytopathology took the initiative to propose recommendations for urinary cytopathology reporting, but these did not receive widespread implementation in practice.

The idea of developing The Paris System for Reporting Urinary Cytopathology was conceived during the International Academy of Cytology Congress held in Paris in May 2013. Drs. Rosenthal and Wojcik have led the Paris System Working Group in this major paradigm shift over the past 2 years, successfully building consensus with input from the international cytopathology and urology communities. Learning from the experience of previous Bethesda systems, The Paris System Working Group appreciated the importance of including international members so that global acceptance of the terminology would be immediately implemented.

Consensus was built by frequent e-mails and conference calls for each of the ten subgroups. The entire Working Group consisted of 49 members, 28 from 12 US states, and 21 from 9 countries including Canada, France, Italy, Japan, Korea, Luxembourg, Slovenia, Switzerland, and the United Kingdom. To involve an international cytology community, the website position statements, posted online by both the International Academy of Cytology and the American Society of Cytopathology, have been translated into Chinese, Korean, and Japanese. Numerous clinical research papers have been presented at national and international meetings to start filling the voids in our global knowledge of the performance of urinary cytology. This explosion of interest in urinary cytology is a direct result of the inauguration of The Paris System. The effort has culminated in the publication of this "Bethesda" type atlas detailing The Paris System's definitions, criteria, and explanatory notes along with corresponding images.

On behalf of the American Society of Cytopathology and the International Academy of Cytology, we are proud to have sponsored this much needed consensus effort and are confident that the adoption and implementation of The Paris System will lead to more uniformity in reporting urinary cytopathology and to improve consistency in patient management.

Chicago, IL, USA Ritu Nayar, M.D.
Northwestern University's Feinberg School of Medicine

Villejuif, France Philippe Vielh, M.D., Ph.D., F.I.A.C.
Gustave Roussy Comprehensive Cancer Center

Prologue

This book is the result of a long-term, determined effort by a group of cytopathologists, cytotechnologists, surgical pathologists, and urologic surgeons dedicated to the definition, description, and codification of urinary specimens. Its importance can be clarified by a brief discussion of issues that have confounded the discipline over the years.

The examination of urine for the diagnosis of human disease is ancient. Its use for the detection of neoplasms of the urinary tract came long before histology. And yet, despite being an integral part of the clinical evaluation of patients with urinary symptomatology, urinary cytology has remained underappreciated. Its perceived weakness, a lack of sensitivity, especially for low-grade tumors in voided urines, has prompted a continual search for ancillary methods.

The perception of a diminished relevance of urinary cytology for the detection of most bladder neoplasms results primarily from two factors: the traditional definition of malignancy, and the insistence of clinicians on labeling all urothelial neoplasms as "bladder cancer." Historically, the concept of malignancy used by most of medicine is derived from gross morphologic concepts predating the twentieth century, where malignancy was diagnosed when tumors showed the life-threatening propensity of local invasion and distant spread. In a slight but important variation, urothelial neoplasms have been considered malignant if they invaded the submucosal tissue or if they recurred. Urothelial malignancy (in contrast to grading) has not been defined on the basis of the degree of anaplasia of the component cells, which, in other systems, is considered a hallmark of malignancy.

Even though it is a conceptual disconnect, it came to pass that lesions composed of cells lacking anaplasia, i.e., cytologic features of malignancy, were classified as carcinomas. Subsequently, clinicians became accustomed to labeling all urothelial neoplasms as "bladder cancer." Urinary cytology, a method that cannot reliably detect tumors when their cells lack anaplasia, was considered deficient. Therefore, attempts to establish exact correlations in nomenclature between histologic and cytologic assessments, although laudable, have foundered largely because the lowest grade urothelial neoplasms are not clinically and morphologically malignant. As stated before, they do not invade and do not show anaplasia. On cytologic examination, these low-grade entities lack features that would make them recognizable as "bladder cancer" in urinary samples. These conceptual problems have tended to marginalize the value of urinary cytopathology in patient care and very likely have contributed to the relative paucity of literature and lack of attempts at standardization of the discipline. The inability of urinary cytopathology to detect nonaggressive lesions that patients are informed are "cancer" has fostered continuous efforts to develop more sensitive techniques, an endeavor that tends to overlook the fact that urinary cytology is currently the only method that can distinguish aggressive, life-threatening carcinomas from noninvasive, indolent lesions.

Many ancillary tests have been developed to detect "bladder cancer," but only a few have been accepted in clinical practice. If applied to specimens composed of morphologically normal cells, all of these ancillary tests achieve the desired increase in sensitivity at the expense of positive predictive value, i.e., diagnostic accuracy, and none can distinguish low-grade, non-aggressive tumors from high-grade, life-threatening carcinomas. None is recommended for routine use by either the American Urological Association or the European Association of Urology.

The perceived weakness of urinary cytology is actually a strength, since low-grade urothelial neoplasms are readily detected by experienced endoscopists, and are not aggressive. In contrast, experienced cytopathologists can detect high-grade carcinomas in adequate samples with a positive predictive value greater than 85 %. Recognition of these lesions is especially beneficial to patients whose bladders may appear endoscopically normal or diffusely nodular after intravesical therapy.

Urinary cytology still remains highly relevant to patient care. It is important for monitoring patients after therapy and is the only noninvasive method that can distinguish low-grade lesions from high-grade urothelial carcinoma. Previous books have tended to be monographs reflecting the research and perspectives of single individuals. This book includes the contributions of international experts representing all facets of the discipline. It is the result of many months of consultation, discussion, and analysis of new and old studies. The Paris System for Reporting Urinary Cytology is an important contribution to patient care; it should be a valuable reference and scientific spring board for the cytopathology community.

Gainesville, FL, USA

William M. Murphy, M.D.
Department of Pathology, Immunology,
and Laboratory Medicine
University of Florida

Abbreviations

AdCa	Adenocarcinoma
AMACR	Alpha-methylacyl-coA racemase
ASC	American Society of Cytopathology
AUC	Atypical urothelial cells
AUTF	Atypical urothelial tissue fragments
BCG	Bacillus Calmette-Guerin
BUTF	Benign urothelial tissue fragments
CAP	College of American Pathologists
CEP	Chromosome enumeration probes
CIS	Carcinoma in situ
CS	CytoSpin™
DAPI	4,6-diamidino, 2-phenylindole dihydrochloride
DS	Direct smear
ERG	ETS-related gene
FDA	U.S. Food and Drug Administration
Fig.	Figure
FISH	Fluorescence in situ hybridization
H&E	Hematoxylin and eosin stain
HGUC	High grade urothelial carcinoma
HPV	Human papillomavirus
IAC	International Academy of Cytology
ISUP	International Society of Urological Pathology
LBP	Liquid-based preparations
LCNEC	Large cell neuroendocrine carcinoma
LGPUC	Low grade papillary urothelial carcinoma
LGPUN	Low grade papillary urothelial neoplasm
LGUC	Low grade urothelial carcinoma
LGUN	Low grade urothelial neoplasia

Stains: All figures are stained by the Papanicolaou method unless otherwise stated.

LSI	Locus specific identifier
mag.	Magnification
N/C	Nuclear to cytoplasmic ratio
NE	Neuroendocrine
NEC	Neuroendocrine carcinoma
NHGUC	Negative for high grade urothelial carcinoma
non-UC	Non-urothelial carcinoma
NOS	Not otherwise specified
PSC	Papanicolaou Society of Cytopathology
PUNLMP	Papillary urothelial neoplasm of low malignant potential
RCC	Renal cell carcinoma
SHGUC	Suspicious for high grade urothelial carcinoma
SMA	Smooth muscle actin
SmCC	Small cell carcinoma
SP	SurePath™ LBP
SqCC	Squamous cell carcinoma
The Paris System	The Paris System for Reporting Urinary Cytology
TP	ThinPrep™
TTF-1	Thyroid transcription factor-1
U-FISH	UroVysion™ fluorescence in situ hybridization
UC	Urothelial carcinoma
UTF	Urothelial tissue fragments
UUT	Upper urinary tract
WHO	World Health Organization

Contents

Editors

Dorothy L. Rosenthal, M.D. Department of Pathology, The Johns Hopkins Hospital, The Johns Hopkins University, Baltimore, MD, USA

Eva M. Wojcik, M.D. Department of Pathology, Loyola University Health Systems, Loyola University, Chicago, IL, USA

Daniel F.I. Kurtycz, M.D. Department of Pathology and Laboratory Medicine, University of Wisconsin School of Medicine and Public Health, Wisconsin State Laboratory of Hygiene, Madison, WI, USA

Contributors

Tatjana Antic, M.D. Department of Pathology, The University of Chicago Medicine, Chicago, IL, USA

Manon Auger, M.D., F.R.C.P.(C) Department of Pathology, McGill University Health Center, Decarie, Montreal, QC, Canada

Güliz A. Barkan, M.D. Department of Pathology, Loyola University Health Systems, Loyola University, Chicago, IL, USA

Trinity J. Bivalacqua, M.D., Ph.D. Department of Urology, The Johns Hopkins Hospital, The Johns Hopkins University, Baltimore, MD, USA

Fadi Brimo, M.D., F.R.C.P.(C) Department of Pathology, Montreal General Hospital, McGill University Health Center, Montreal, QC, Canada

Lukas Bubendorf, M.D. Institute of Pathology, University Hospital Basel, Basel, Switzerland

Nancy P. Caraway, M.D. Department of Pathology, The University of Texas MD Anderson Cancer Center, Houston, TX, USA

Ashish Chandra, M.D., F.R.C.Path., Dip.R.C.Path. (Cytol) Department of Cellular Pathology, Guy's & St Thomas' NHS Foundation Trust, London, England, UK

Michael B. Cohen, M.D. Department of Pathology, University of Utah Health Sciences Center, Salt Lake City, UT, USA

Monique Courtade-Saïdi, M.D., Ph.D. Pathology and Histology-Cytology Department, Toulouse-Rangueil University Hospital, Toulouse University Cancer Institute, Toulouse, France

William N. Crabtree, Ph.D., S.C.T. (A.S.C.P.) Department of Pathology and Laboratory Medicine, Indiana University Health Pathology Laboratory, Indiana University School of Medicine, Indianapolis, IN, USA

Tarik M. Elsheikh, M.D. Department of Pathology, Pathology and Laboratory Medicine Institute, Cleveland Clinic, Cleveland, OH, USA

Guido Fadda, M.D. Division of Anatomic Pathology and Histology, Agostino Gemelli School of Medicine, Catholic University of the Sacred Heart, Rome, Italy

Andrew H. Fischer, M.D. Department of Pathology and Cell Biology, University of Massachusetts Memorial Medical Center, Worcester, MA, USA

Margareta Strojan Fležar, M.D., Ph.D. Institute of Pathology, University of Ljubljana, Ljubljana, Slovenia

Gary W. Gill, C.T. (A.S.C.P.) Cyto-Logics, Inc., Indianapolis, IN, USA

Hui Guan, M.D., Ph.D. Department of Pathology, Harper University Hospital, Detroit Medical Center, Wayne State University Medical School, Detroit, MI, USA

Jee-Young Han, M.D., Ph.D. Department of Pathology, Inha University Hospital, Incheon, South Korea

Rana S. Hoda, M.D. Department of Pathology, New York Presbyterian Hospital, Weill Cornell Medical College, New York, NY, USA

Ashish M. Kamat, M.D. Department of Urology, The University of Texas MD Anderson Cancer Center, Houston, TX, USA

Ruth L. Katz, M.D., M.B.B.C.H. Department of Pathology, MD Anderson Cancer Center, The University of Texas, Houston, TX, USA

Deidra P. Kelly, C.T. (A.S.C.P.) Department of Pathology, Johns Hopkins Hospital, Baltimore, MD, USA

Mitsuru Kinjo, M.D., Ph.D. Department of Laboratory Medicine, Steel Memorial Yawata Hospital, Kitakyushu, Fukuoka, Japan

Zulfia McCroskey, M.D. Department of Pathology, Loyola University Health Systems, Loyola University, Chicago, IL, USA

Sachiko Minamiguchi, M.D., Ph.D. Department of Diagnostic Pathology, Kyoto University Hospital, Kyoto, Japan

Hiroshi Ohtani, M.D., Ph.D. Department of Pathology, Hakujyuji Hospital, Fukuoka, Japan

Matthew T. Olson, M.D. Department of Pathology, The Johns Hopkins Hospital, The Johns Hopkins University, Baltimore, MD, USA

Christopher L. Owens, M.D. Department of Pathology, University of Massachusetts Memorial Medical Center, Worcester, MA, USA

Stefan E. Pambuccian, M.D. Department of Pathology, Loyola University Health Systems, Loyola University, Chicago, IL, USA

Eric Piaton, M.D., Ph.D. Hospices Civils de Lyon, Centre de Pathologie Est, Hôpital Femme-Mère-Enfant, Bron, Université Claude Bernard Lyon 1, Lyon, France

Spasenija Savic Prince, M.D. Institute of Pathology, University Hospital Basel, Basel, Switzerland

Marcus L. Quek, M.D. Department of Urology, Loyola University Health Systems, Loyola University, Chicago, IL, USA

Jae Y. Ro, M.D., Ph.D. Department of Pathology and Genomic Medicine, Houston Methodist Hospital, Weill Medical College of Cornell University, Houston, TX, USA

Department of Pathology, The University of Texas MD Anderson Cancer Center, Houston, TX, USA

Department of Pathology, Yonsei and Ewha Womans University Hospitals, Seoul, South Korea

Fernando Schmitt, M.D., Ph.D. Laboratoire National de Santé, Luxembourg City, Luxembourg

Mark P. Schoenberg, M.D. Department of Urology, Montefiore Medical Center, Albert Einstein College of Medicine of Yeshiva University, Bronx, NY, USA

Tatsuro Shimokama, M.D., Ph.D. Division of Anatomic Pathology, Steel Memorial Yawata Hospital, Kitakyushu, Fukuoka, Japan

Taizo Shiraishi, M.D., Ph.D. Department of Oncologic Pathology, Institute of Medical Life Sciences, Mie University Graduate School, Mie, Japan

Momin T. Siddiqui, M.D. Department of Pathology and Laboratory Medicine, Emory University School of Medicine, Atlanta, GA, USA

Sun Hee Sung, M.D., Ph.D. Department of Pathology, MokDong Hospital, Ewha Womans University, Seoul, South Korea

Z. Laura Tabatabai, M.D. Department of Pathology, University of California San Francisco, San Francisco, CA, USA

Rosemary H. Tambouret, M.D. Department of Pathology, Massachusetts General Hospital, Harvard Medical School, Boston, MA, USA

Yuji Tokuda, M.D., Ph.D. Department of Urology, Saga University, Saga, Japan

Toyonori Tsuzuki, M.D., Ph.D. Department of Pathology, Japanese Red Cross Nagoya Daini Hospital, Nagoya, Japan

Christopher J. VandenBussche, M.D., Ph.D. Department of Pathology, The Johns Hopkins Hospital, The Johns Hopkins University, Baltimore, MD, USA

Theodorus H. Van der Kwast, M.D., Ph.D., F.R.C.P.(C) Department of Laboratory Medicine and Pathobiology, Toronto General Hospital, University of Toronto, Toronto, ON, Canada

Philippe Vielh, M.D., Ph.D. Department of Biopathology, Gustave Roussy Comprehensive Cancer Center, Villejuif, France

Chapter 1
Pathogenesis of Urothelial Carcinoma

Eva M. Wojcik and Stefan E. Pambuccian

Background

For any reporting system to be successful and be applied in daily practice, it must be based on consensus, evidence, inclusion, acceptance, and understanding [1]. Anyone using the reporting scheme should have an opportunity to take part in its creation and verification. In addition, important principles that have to be followed are the understanding of the disease, or entity, that the reporting system applies to, and the clinical implications of the proposed diagnostic categories.

The main goal of urinary cytology is the detection of urothelial carcinoma that is clinically significant, namely high-grade urothelial carcinoma (HGUC). Therefore, the understanding of this disease, and particularly its pathogenesis, was crucial in the process of creating The Paris System for Reporting Urinary Cytology (The Paris System).

Two Pathways of Neoplastic Transformation of Urothelium

For many years it has been known that urothelial carcinoma has two distinct pathogenetic pathways [2–12], a hyperplasia pathway and a dysplasia pathway, a simplified overview of which is shown in Fig. 1.1. An additional hyperplasia/dysplasia pathway has been recently proposed by some authors [12, 13], but, for the sake of simplicity, we have combined this putative third pathway that shows the molecular abnormalities of both the hyperplasia and the dysplasia pathway, i.e., both fibroblast growth factor receptor 3 (FGFR3) and p53 gene (TP53) abnormalities, with the dysplasia pathway. The hyperplasia pathway is more common, accounting for about 80 % of cases, and starts with urothelial hyperplasia that progresses to low-grade papillary urothelial carcinoma (LGUC). One of the very first molecular changes seen in the development of LGUC is the deletion of the gene CDKN2A

D.L. Rosenthal et al. (eds.), *The Paris System for Reporting Urinary Cytology*,
DOI 10.1007/978-3-319-22864-8_1

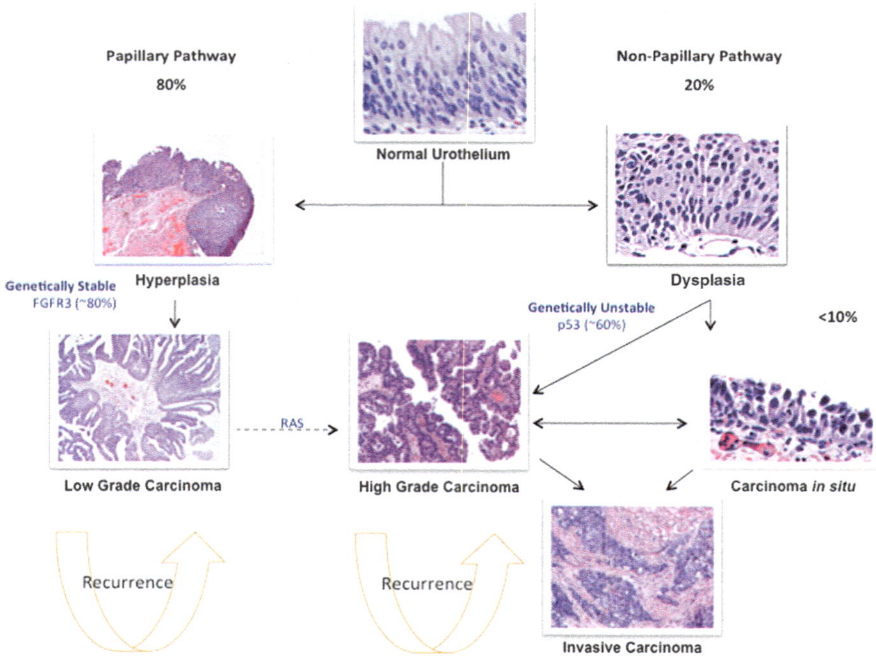

Fig. 1.1 Schematic representation of the two major pathways of urothelial carcinogenesis: Note that while recurrences are common in both pathways, invasive disease is seen only in the dysplasia pathway (HGUC); the *dotted line* represents a questionable transition pathway from LGUC to HGUC

(cyclin-dependent kinase inhibitor 2A), located on the short arm of chromosome 9, which encodes the p16^{INK4A} protein. This pathway is genetically stable and is characterized by FGFR3 alterations, especially activating point mutations in FGFR3, which is detected in over 80 % of LGUC [12]. These tumors are characterized by a high recurrence rate, but otherwise nonaggressive behavior [14].

The second pathway, the dysplasia pathway, is less frequent and is responsible for the formation of approximately 20 % of urothelial carcinomas. This pathway leads to high-grade urothelial tumors. It starts with dysplasia, which progresses either to the formation of a high-grade papillary tumor or, in a smaller percentage of cases, to flat urothelial carcinoma (carcinoma in situ). HGUC is also associated with a high recurrence rate but, most importantly, has a high risk of progression to muscle-invasive, stage T2, T3, and T4 tumors with lymph node and systemic metastases. This pathway is genetically unstable and is associated with a number of additional mutations; the most significant of them are inactivating mutations of TP53, which are seen in approximately 60 % of these tumors.

What is of significance is that the key molecular abnormalities associated with the dysplasia pathway, especially the TP53 mutations, which are strongly associated with high-grade and high-stage urothelial carcinomas, are essentially mutually exclusive with the molecular abnormalities characterizing the hyperplasia pathway [13].

It was historically believed that at some point of the hyperplasia pathway, LGUC will acquire more mutations, particularly RAS mutations, and will progress to HGUC [15]. In general, the accepted rate of progression was about 10 %. However, there are recent studies demonstrating that noninvasive LGUC (Ta) has a very low risk of progression (less than 1–5 %) [16]. In addition, RAS (HRAS and KRAS) mutations, that were believed to be necessary for the progression to high-grade tumors, are mutually exclusive with the FGFR3 mutations that are characteristic for the low-grade pathway [12]. This could potentially indicate that these two pathways are completely separate from each other. If that would prove to be right, low-grade carcinoma and high-grade carcinoma may represent two entirely different diseases. This finding would potentially be of great clinical significance, considering that there are already opinions that low-grade tumors originating from the hyperplasia pathway should not even be called "carcinoma". All these pathogenetic considerations aside, truly clinically significant urothelial neoplasms are the ones that have the ability to invade deep muscle; these are HGUC.

Therefore, the guiding principle for The Paris System is to detect HGUC. In line with this principle, the negative category includes reactive changes, infectious and nonneoplastic conditions, as well as cases that may have some cytologic features of low-grade urothelial neoplasms, but are negative for HGUC. Therefore, the proposed diagnostic category is "Negative for High-Grade Urothelial Carcinoma" (NHGUC). Despite the fact that we strive to detect all high-grade urothelial tumors, we recognize that there will be cases where the definite diagnosis cannot be made. Therefore, in The Paris System we include the categories of "Atypical Urothelial Cells" (AUC) and "Suspicious for High-Grade Urothelial Carcinoma" (SHGUC). Of importance is the understanding that the difference between the two categories, suspicious for HGUC and positive for HGUC, are quantitative since the diagnostic features for these two categories are based on similar morphologic findings.

Although the diagnosis of LGUC is not the main goal of this system, a separate diagnostic category has been included to define those circumstances where cytologic features of low-grade urothelial neoplasms (LGUN) are present (see Chap. 7). We recognize that the cytologic diagnosis of LGUC can be rarely made, and should be based only on the presence of well-defined fibrovascular cores in the absence of cellular atypia. Otherwise, if there is a high cytologic suspicion for a low-grade lesion and/or there is a papillary lesion present on cystoscopy and/or biopsy, a diagnosis of LGUN can be included in the overall Negative for HGUC category with a secondary diagnosis of LGUN.

References

1. Ali SZ, Leteurtre E. The official nomenclature and terminologies in diagnostic cytopathology: history, evolution, applicability and future. Ann Pathol. 2012;32:e3–7. 389–93.
2. Koss LG. Bladder cancer from a perspective of 40 years. J Cell Biochem Suppl. 1992;16I:23–9.

3. Spruck III CH, Ohneseit PF, Gonzalez-Zulueta M, et al. Two molecular pathways to transitional cell carcinoma of the bladder. Cancer Res. 1994;54:784–8.
4. Wu XR. Urothelial tumorigenesis: a tale of divergent pathways. Nat Rev Cancer. 2005;5:713–25.
5. Knowles MA. Molecular subtypes of bladder cancer: Jekyll and Hyde or chalk and cheese? Carcinogenesis. 2006;27:361–73.
6. Cordon-Cardo C. Molecular alterations associated with bladder cancer initiation and progression. Scand J Urol Nephrol Suppl. 2008;218:154–65.
7. Castillo-Martin M, Domingo-Domenech J, Karni-Schmidt O, Matos T, Cordon-Cardo C. Molecular pathways of urothelial development and bladder tumorigenesis. Urol Oncol. 2010;28:401–8.
8. Pollard C, Smith SC, Theodorescu D. Molecular genesis of non-muscle-invasive urothelial carcinoma (NMIUC). Expert Rev Mol Med. 2010;12:e10.
9. Cheng L, Zhang S, MacLennan GT, Williamson SR, Lopez-Beltran A, Montironi R. Bladder cancer: translating molecular genetic insights into clinical practice. Hum Pathol. 2011;42:455–81.
10. Al Hussain TO, Akhtar M. Molecular basis of urinary bladder cancer. Adv Anat Pathol. 2013;20:53–60.
11. Netto GJ. Molecular genetics and genomics progress in urothelial bladder cancer. Semin Diagn Pathol. 2013;30:313–20.
12. Knowles MA, Hurst CD. Molecular biology of bladder cancer: new insights into pathogenesis and clinical diversity. Nat Rev Cancer. 2015;15:25–41.
13. Seront E, Machiels JP. Molecular biology and targeted therapies for urothelial carcinoma. Cancer Treat Rev. 2015;41:341–53.
14. Amin MB, Smith SC, Reuter VE, et al. Update for the practicing pathologist: the international consultation on urologic disease—European Association of Urology consultation on bladder cancer. Mod Pathol. 2015;28:612–30.
15. Shinohara N, Koyanagi T. Ras signal transduction in carcinogenesis and progression of bladder cancer: molecular target for treatment? Urol Res. 2002;30:273–81.
16. Nielsen ME, Smith AB, Meyer AM, et al. Trends in stage-specific incidence rates for urothelial carcinoma of the bladder in the United States: 1988 to 2006. Cancer. 2014;120:86–95.

Chapter 2
Adequacy of Urine Specimens (Adequacy)

Matthew T. Olson, Güliz A. Barkan, Monique Courtade-Saïdi, Z. Laura Tabatabai, Yuji Tokuda, Toyonori Tsuzuki, and Christopher J. VandenBussche

Introduction

Adequacy is a source of disagreement and controversy in all areas of cytopathology, and urinary tract specimens are no exception. In fact, it is one of the most common causes of diagnostic discrepancy when two pathologists interpret the same cytology specimen [1]. Unlike other systems in diagnostic cytology, however, urine analysis is the result of a complex interplay between numerous human and laboratory variables. The variables related to cytological preservation and preparation are not entirely standardized beyond a widespread use of cytological preservatives and preparation devices from a few commercial providers. At least three other pre-analytical specimen variables may influence the performance characteristics of urinary tract cytology and may confound adequacy determination: collection type, cellularity, and volume. Thus, to address adequacy properly, each of these variables must be considered in the context of all the others. Herein lies the pith of recommendations for adequacy evaluation from The Paris System for Reporting Urinary Cytology (The Paris System).

Adequacy is an essential discussion for cytopathologists because cytology specimens are generally, incorrectly perceived to have low negative predictive value. This is due to several factors, and chief among them is the unavoidable limitation of making diagnostic inferences based on a limited sampling of cellular material. To frame the sampling of the urinary tract numerically, a healthy average maximally distended human bladder has an approximate value of 600 mL. Approximating a spherical shape, the inner surface area of that bladder would be approximately 350 cm^2 (350×10^{-4} m^2). The average urothelial cell has an approximate diameter of 20 µm or a two-dimensional surface area of 314 µm^2 (314×10^{-12} m^2). The urothelium is about five cells thick, so the total number of urothelial cells lining the bladder is on the order of 10^8–10^9 cells. Thus, even a highly cellular urine specimen contains an infinitesimally small fraction of the urothelial cells lining the bladder, and may contain no or very few abnormal cells.

D.L. Rosenthal et al. (eds.), *The Paris System for Reporting Urinary Cytology*,
DOI 10.1007/978-3-319-22864-8_2

When considered this way, a false negative result is the stochastically inevitable byproduct of an inherently limited sampling size. Because variation in sampling size exists among urinary tract samples, we must determine the number of benign cells present for examination in order to confidently claim that the remaining urothelium is benign as well.

The Adequacy Algorithm

For the purposes of this chapter, the term "adequacy" is used to refer to the usefulness of the specimen to diagnose or broach the suspicion of urothelial carcinoma. As such, a specimen taken in the context of acute bacterial cystitis that shows only neutrophils may be inadequate for the evaluation of urothelial carcinoma but perfectly adequate to answer a specific non-oncologic clinical question. Adequacy of urine specimens for the diagnosis of urothelial carcinoma is determined by the interplay of four specimen characteristics: collection type, cellularity, volume, and cytomorphological findings. Of these, cytomorphological findings should be considered first, since the presence of any atypical, suspicious, or malignant findings makes a specimen intrinsically adequate regardless of the collection type, cellularity, or volume. Thus, a decision about specimen adequacy is most relevant when there are no findings indicative of a disease process. In that case, the other specimen characteristics—collection type, cellularity, and volume—should factor into the classification of adequacy.

Given the current state of urinary cytology practice, publications on the role and specific qualifiers of collection type, cellularity, and volume are limited and the opinions expressed in these publications are variable. This impedes the development of evidence-based consensus guidelines. Thus, adequacy recommendations for The Paris System are centered around an adequacy algorithm shown in Fig. 2.1. The purpose of this algorithm is threefold. The first is to communicate the relationship that exists among collection type, cellularity, and volume in The Paris System. The second purpose is to guide individual laboratories in validating appropriate cut-offs for their own practice settings at each branch in the adequacy algorithm. Finally, the ultimate purpose is to frame all future investigations dealing with adequacy of urine specimens so that each decision point will have a clear evidence basis supporting consensus cut-offs for volume and cellularity in the context of the collection type.

The adequacy algorithm does not currently take into consideration the method used for preparing urinary tract specimens. This is intentional given the incomplete nature of evidence on this topic (see Chap. 10). Based on the established differences in gynecological cytopathology adequacy criteria, which depend on specimen preparation type, we expect to see preparation-dependent cut-offs at each point in the algorithm. However, the generic approach to adequacy should be uniform regardless of the specimen preparation method used in any particular laboratory.

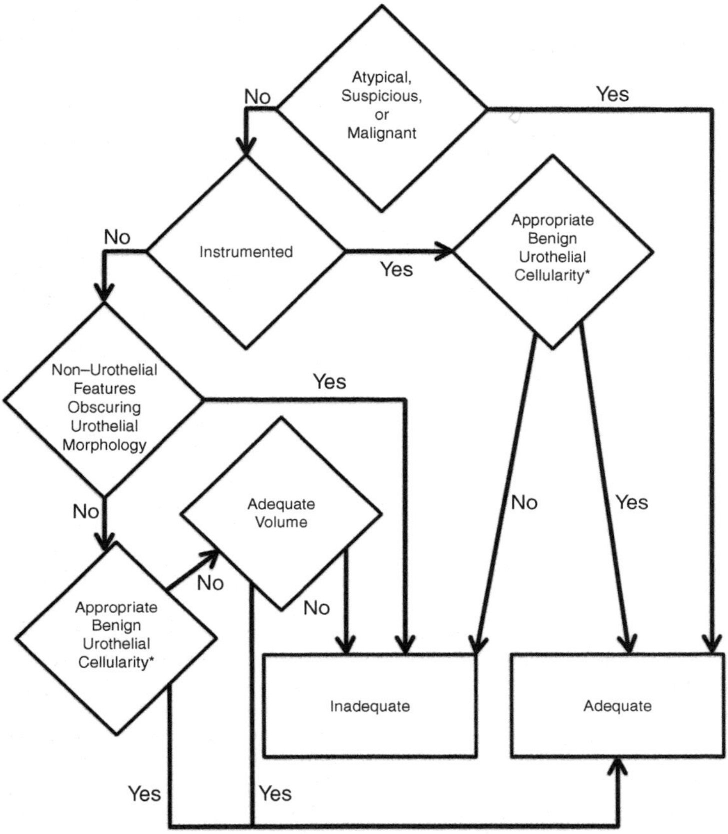

Fig. 2.1 The adequacy algorithm shows The Paris System's recommendation for the proper relationship between specimen source, cytological diagnosis, urine volume, urothelial cellularity, and obscuring features. Obscuring features include non-urothelial cells such as vaginal contaminants, bacteria, acute inflammation, sperm, and crystals which, when copious, may obscure the finding and characterization of urothelial cells. "*": Cut-offs for appropriate benign urothelial cellularity should be validated for both instrumented and non-instrumented sources

Volume and Adequacy

There is a common misperception that cells in body fluids are solutes in a homogenous solution. However, urine is a heterogeneous mixture of non-solute particulates: crystals, microorganisms, decaying cell remnants, and cells. It is heterogeneous because the particulates are not evenly distributed throughout the volume. Cells are denser than most aqueous solutions, so they sink. If only the supernatant, which is acellular or paucicellular, is examined because the first drops of a urine stream were not captured in the specimen container or because the specimen was inadvertently decanted, the results will be suboptimal.

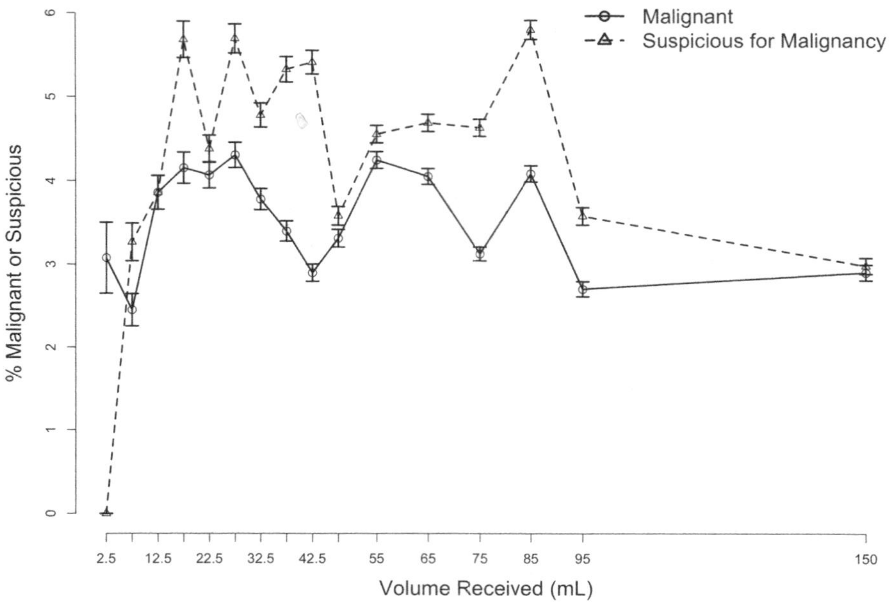

Fig. 2.2 Relationship of volume to the prevalence of malignant and suspicious diagnosis for demographically comparable populations. There were no suspicious samples in the lowest volume bin, and there was a nearly linear increase in the suspicious fraction up to the bin centered on 15 mL. A specimen was nearly twofold more likely to be suspicious when more than 15 mL was received than when less than 5 mL was received. The global maximum for the malignancy fraction was seen at 27.5 mL (range: 25–30 mL) which was also the location of a local maximum for the suspicious fraction. The global maximum for the suspicious curve was centered at 85 mL, and the difference between the global maximum (5.8, 95 % CI: 5.6–5.9) and the local maximum at 27.5 mL (5.7, 95 % CI: 5.5–5.9) was not statistically significant. Based on this analysis, we concluded that at least 30 mL are necessary to consider a urine specimen fully adequate when processed with SurePath (From VandenBussche et al. [2] with kind permission of John Wiley & Sons) Copyright © 1999-2015 John Wiley & Sons, Inc.

Volume-only factors into the adequacy of urine specimens for voided urines in the urinary tract adequacy algorithm for obvious reasons—instrumented specimens have artificial volumes, and their adequacy is based on operator skill and measured by cellularity. Conversely urine volume is important for voided urines for two main reasons (Fig. 2.2). First, in at least one study [2] there is a clear correlation between low-volume specimens and the lack of malignant diagnoses, suggesting that some benign diagnoses in small-volume specimens are due to undersampling of the potential voided urine volume rather than an absence of disease. This phenomenon is well known in effusion cytology, a field in which there can be up to a fivefold difference in the malignancy prevalence that is only explainable on the basis of the volume submitted to the laboratory. Second, the volume received by a laboratory can be evidence of specimen manipulation at some point in the collection. In a single study, the data suggests that a cut-off of 30 mL is appropriate in a laboratory that uses SurePath® preparation performed on fresh unfixed voided urines [2].

While volume is an important factor in the adequacy algorithm for voided urines, it is clearly not a variable that should disqualify a specimen from analysis a priori. Doing so would lead to the discarding of low-volume specimens in which diagnostic findings may be present. Two microscope-dependent nodes precede volume in the adequacy algorithm: the finding of atypical, suspicious, or malignant cells or the finding of an adequate number of benign urothelial cells. The exact number has yet to be determined rigorously. Further, as the urothelial content can only be approximated with current technology prior to processing the specimen and examining it, laboratories should not reject urine specimens based on volume alone.

Adequacy of Instrumented Urinary Tract Cytology Specimens

Instrumented urinary tract specimens are forced exfoliative specimens that include urinary bladder washing specimens—occasionally called "barbotage" specimens. Other instrumented urinary specimens are washings and brushings from the urethra, ureters, and renal pelvis. Of these, the specimen type most commonly processed in most laboratories is the bladder washing [3].

The cellularity of instrumented urinary tract specimens may be affected by various technical factors, including those related to the cystoscopists' skill, method of performing the washing, amount of fluid with which the bladder is washed, and the distance of the cystoscope to the mucosa. While it may not be possible to control these factors, setting adequacy criteria will alert the clinicians that the specimen has insufficient cellularity and may therefore be more prone to a false negative diagnosis.

Compared with voided urine specimens, bladder washing specimens have a volume dependent on the amount of fluid instilled into the bladder, lack contamination with non-urothelial cells, and usually have a higher cellularity. These features may be responsible for their higher sensitivity [4] but also suggest the need for volume-independent adequacy criteria. Quantitative adequacy criteria based on specimen cellularity have been established for Pap tests [5] and thyroid aspirates [6] based on evidence obtained by studies using serial dilutions [5] or by retrospective review of cytology specimens with surgical excision follow-up [6]. To date, only a single study has applied both methods to bladder wash specimens in order to establish cell count adequacy criteria for bladder wash specimens that have been processed with the ThinPrep method [7]. In that study, an adequate bladder barbotage specimen was determined to have at least 20 well-preserved, well-visualized urothelial cells per 10 high-power fields. This cut-off was only viable in the absence of obscuring features. The presence of excessive and obscuring lubricant, inflammatory cells, or red blood cells obscuring the urothelial cells should be interpreted as "unsatisfactory/nondiagnostic". In specimens where there are 10–20 well-preserved, well-visualized urothelial cells per 10 high-power fields "satisfactory but limited by low cellularity", and in specimens where <10 well-preserved, well-visualized urothelial cells per 10 high-power fields "unsatisfactory/nondiagnostic" diagnoses are appropriate. Given that these thresholds were developed using ThinPrep, additional studies should be pursued for the other specimen preparation methods. Similarly, since the studies have been performed on bladder washing specimens, the adequacy criteria for voided specimens are not rigorously defined. As data become available on these specimens, the criteria will reflect the evidence, and this evidence can lend hard quantitative data to the adequacy algorithm.

The Less-Than-Optimal Adequacy Category

The most uncertain feature of the adequacy algorithm is the classification of voided urine specimens that lack appropriate numbers of benign urothelial cells but have an adequate volume. There is currently no evidence supporting or disproving a need for the demonstration of benign urothelial cells in voided urine specimens. In many practices, specimens that meet every adequacy criteria except for urothelial cellularity are assigned a "less-than-optimal" adequacy. While the data are small and limited to a subset of a single institutional experience, the use of this category appears to be useful; patients returning to provide a repeat voided urine sample usually yielded fully adequate specimens, some of which have diagnostic findings [2].

Recommendations

Adequacy in urine specimens is a topic for which there is little concrete quality data. As such, the recommendations for adequacy in The Paris System center on the adequacy algorithm. When properly validated for each decision node, this algorithm will increase standardization and quality in reporting across laboratories. As the quantitative results of validation become available in the literature, we expect this algorithm to adopt more defined prescriptive qualities that will lead to uniform practice in all urine adequacy determinations.

References

1. Olson MT, Boonyaarunnate T, Aragon Han P, Umbricht CB, Ali SZ, Zeiger MA. A tertiary center's experience with second review of 3885 thyroid cytopathology specimens. J Clin Endocrinol Metab. 2013;98:1450–7.
2. VandenBussche CJ, Rosenthal DL, Olson MT. A minimum volume of 30 mL is necessary to ensure that a voided urine specimen is benign: a retrospective review of 15,731 cases. Cancer Cytopathol. DOI: 10.1002/cncy.21634 and PubMed ID: 26524350.
3. Barkan GA, Tabatabai ZL, Sturgis C, Kurtycz DF, Souers RJ, Nayar R. In preparation for The Paris System for Reporting Urinary Tract Cytopathology (TPSRUTC): observations from the

2014 supplemental questionnaire of the College of American Pathologists (CAP) Cytopathology Interlaboratory Comparison Program (CICP) (abstract). Lab Invest. 2015;95 Suppl 1:83A.
4. Murphy WM, Crabtree WN, Jukkola AF, Soloway MS. The diagnostic value of urine versus bladder washing in patients with bladder cancer. J Urol. 1981;126:320–2.
5. Studeman KD, Ioffe OB, Puszkiewicz J, Sauvegeot J, Henry MR. Effect of cellularity on the sensitivity of detecting squamous lesions in liquid-based cervical cytology. Acta Cytol. 2003;47:605–10.
6. Michael CW, Pang Y, Pu RT, Hasteh F, Griffith KA. Cellular adequacy for thyroid aspirates prepared by ThinPrep: how many cells are needed? Diagn Cytopathol. 2007;35:792–7.
7. Prather J, Arville B, Chatt G, Pambuccian SE, Wojcik EM, Quek ML, Barkan GA. Evidence-based adequacy criteria for urinary bladder barbotage cytology. J Am Soc Cytopathol. 2015;4:57–62.

Chapter 3
Negative for High-Grade Urothelial Carcinoma (Negative)

Dorothy L. Rosenthal, Michael B. Cohen, Hui Guan, Christopher L. Owens, Yuji Tokuda, and Eva M. Wojcik

Background

Many cytology reporting systems regard the "Negative" category as containing only normal cells from the particular body site without any alterations. Any other mild changes are placed in the "atypical category". If the Working Group for The Paris System followed that premise, the "atypical category" would be so large that it would serve no clinical usefulness [1].

Following the lead of The Bethesda System for Reporting Gynecologic Cytology, The Paris System includes in the negative category all entities that pose no significant risk to the patient for developing HGUC based upon available studies. Therefore, if a specific cause of a particular morphologic alteration in urothelial cells is recognized and the cause is not associated with malignancy, e.g., radiation-induced "atypia", those cases are best classified as "Negative for HGUC" and not atypical, unless there are other cellular alterations in the sample that warrant the atypical designation. Furthermore, the goal of The Paris System is to highlight those cases that are at risk for HGUC. Therefore, the Negative for High-Grade Urothelial Carcinoma (NHGUC) category emphasizes that goal by stating "Negative for High-Grade Urothelial Carcinoma".

A recent publication [2] reviewed those entities that cause discernible cytologic changes but pose no threat of neoplasia to the patient. This chapter includes those morphologic entities with non-neoplastic phenotypic changes. Those entities in which there may be an association with neoplasia will be so noted and included in both the negative and atypical categories with appropriate codicils.

1. Benign cytologic changes
    (a) Benign/reactive urothelial cells, squamous, and glandular cells
    (b) True tissue fragments and clusters without morphologic changes in the absence of instrumentation and after instrumentation
    (c) Alterations caused by urinary bladder and renal calculi

D.L. Rosenthal et al. (eds.), *The Paris System for Reporting Urinary Cytology*,
DOI 10.1007/978-3-319-22864-8_3

(d) Viral cytopathic effect, especially polyoma (BK) virus, unless accompanied by atypical cells
(e) Post-treatment effect of bladder instillations, especially BCG
(f) Post-treatment effect for non-bladder disease, e.g., pelvic irradiation for other malignancies; systemic chemotherapy that may affect the urothelium, e.g., cyclophosphamide
(g) Enteric epithelium following a surgical urinary diversion post-cystectomy
(h) Unexpected normal cells, e.g., sperm, seminal vesicle cells, cells from the female genital tract

2. Use of ancillary tests to confirm causative agent, if history does not provide clinical correlation

Definition of Negative for High-Grade Urothelial Carcinoma

A sample of urine, either voided or instrumented, may be considered benign, i.e., NHGUC, if any of the following components are present in the specimen:

- Benign urothelial, glandular, and squamous cells
- Benign urothelial tissue fragments (BUTF) and urothelial sheets or clusters
- Changes associated with lithiasis
- Viral cytopathic effect; polyoma virus (BK virus—decoy cells)
- Post-therapy effect, including epithelial cells from urinary diversions

Criteria of Components of NHGUC

Benign Superficial (Umbrella) Urothelial Cells

The designation of "benign/reactive superficial (umbrella, cap, or dome) urothelial cells" applies to a urine specimen that is adequate for evaluation and consists of large superficial urothelial cells (Fig. 3.1a–c).

Fig. 3.1 Superficial urothelial (umbrella) cells. (**a**) The cytoplasm of large superficial cells is very frothy and abundant resulting in a low N/C ratio. Nuclei have pale finely granular chromatin. Nucleoli can be prominent, but don't reflect any abnormality. Multinucleation is common, especially in instrumented samples (*Washing, TP, medium mag*). (**b**) In addition to superficial (umbrella) cells, clusters of smaller cells are seen (*arrows*). The nuclei are darker and slightly smaller than in superficial cells but the nuclear shapes are round, nuclear membranes are smooth, and architecture is uniform. N/C ratios are high due to the small amount of cytoplasm of each cell (*Washing, TP, medium mag*). (**c**) These true tissue fragments (TTF) clearly illustrate the image of "umbrella" cells. By definition, they are the most superficial cells in the bladder, creating an "Umbrella" over all other urothelial cells. Their nuclear and cytoplasmic character is the same as other superficial cells, but additionally, they possess a thickened cytoplasmic edge that doesn't go all around the cell. This constitutes the asymmetric unit membrane, providing a barrier between the toxic urine and the blood (*Washing, CS, medium mag*)

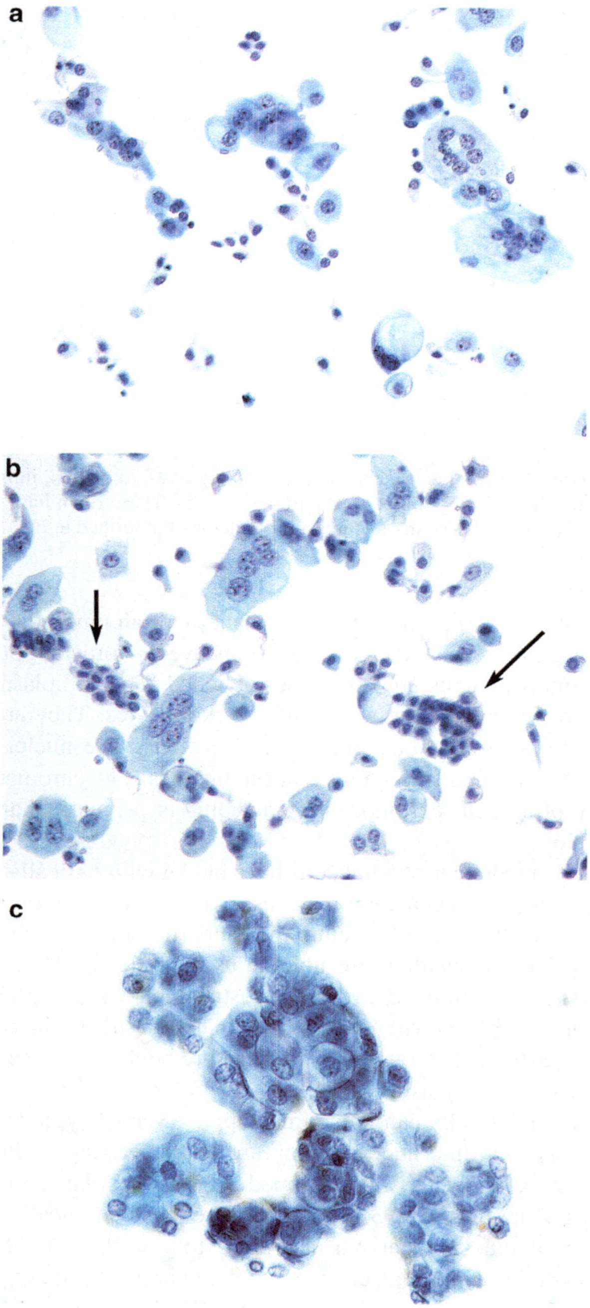
a
b
c

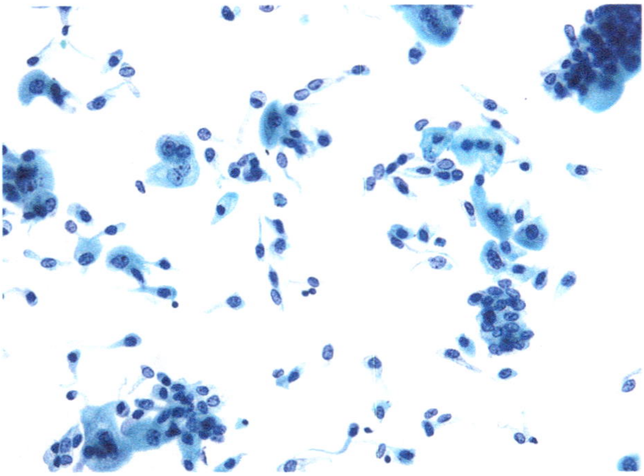

Fig. 3.2 Intermediate urothelial cells. The intermediate layer of urothelium, immediately underneath the umbrella cells, is easily dissociated into single cells. These often have cells with cytoplasmic (cercariaform) tails (All of the features are normal, and described in Fig. 3.1b.) (*Washing, TP, medium mag.*)

Superficial cells are large, shaped like the canopy of an umbrella, with rounded (convex) luminal surfaces and scalloped (concaved) borders onto which the underlying intermediate cells are sometimes attached. The cytoplasm is abundant and vacuolated or foamy, not to be mistaken as koilocytes. They are often bi- or multinucleated, or may contain a single large nucleus. The nuclei are centrally located, round to oval, with smooth nuclear membranes. The chromatin is fine and an occasionally prominent chromocenter/nucleolus is present. Characteristically, the N/C ratio is low.

In contrast, intermediate urothelial cells have nuclei with basically the same size and character as superficial cells, but have less cytoplasm, imparting a higher N/C ratio (Fig. 3.2). Since they are less mature than superficial cells, their nuclear chromatin may be a bit coarser than the ubiquitous superficial cells, but thin, even nuclear membranes and uniform chromatin distribution will support their totally benign condition. Cytoplasm will not be as vacuolated as superficial cells, but is not completely opaque (homogeneous), the latter feature being cited as a characteristic of low-grade urothelial neoplasms [3–6].

Although superficial cells can sometimes appear very "atypical" by virtue of enlarged nuclei and multiple nucleoli, they are recognized as benign/reactive by their low N/C ratio, characteristic scalloped edges, vacuolated cytoplasm, and smooth nuclear membranes (Fig. 3.3a, b). Even the most "atypical" umbrella cells do not justify the diagnosis of atypia in urine cytology. What is of significance, however, is the fact that umbrella cells may contain abnormal amounts of DNA [7] and may be a potential pitfall in any ancillary tests that are based upon DNA ploidy, including fluorescence in situ hybridization (FISH) [8–10]. A reason for the "reactive" changes should be sought, either from clinical history, or from the sample itself, e.g., neutrophils, fungi, calculi.

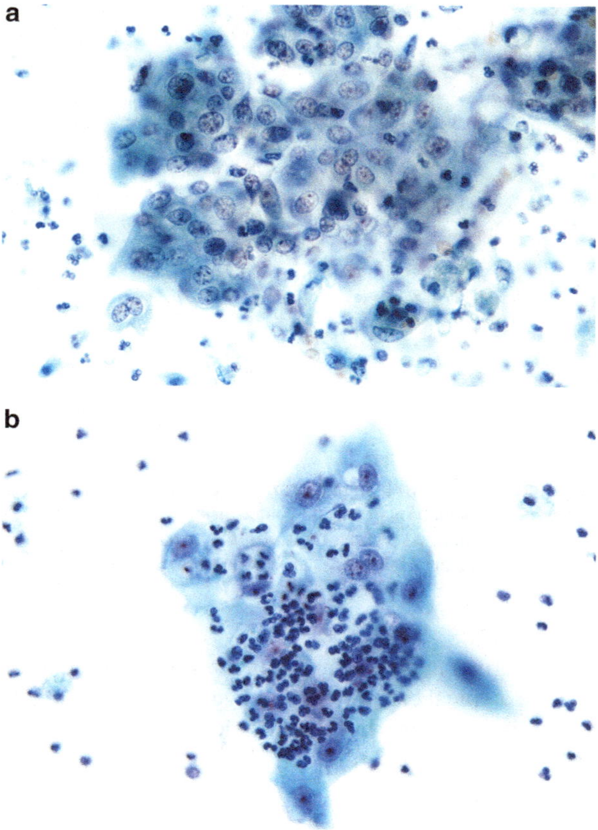

Fig. 3.3 Reactive umbrella cells. (**a**) Most inflamed epithelial cells demonstrate changes, especially in the nuclei. Nucleoli may become prominent, but nuclear chromatin will remain finely granular and shapes will remain round. The cytoplasm retains its transparency. Neutrophils will ordinarily be the inflammatory cells, but lymphocytes may be present if a chronic process is ongoing (*Washing, CS, medium mag.*). (**b**) Changes consistent with epithelial repair are identical with those in all other body sites. The epithelium appears stretched (like Turkish taffy) but all cells stay connected, retaining their intercellular connections. Inflammatory cells pepper the TTF (*Washing, TP, medium mag.*)

Squamous Epithelial Cells, Both Superficial and Intermediate

Both men and women can be expected to have benign squamous cells (Fig. 3.4) in their urine, although they are much more common in women. In voided urine from a woman, the origin is usually the urethra but may be a contaminant from the vagina or perineum. If the sample is instrumented, then the origin is either the urethra or the bladder trigone in both men and women. Of note, chronic irritation, particularly due to stones, can cause squamous metaplasia leading to presence of squamous cells in instrumented urines. Squamous cells can arise from the trigone secondary to hormonal influence and resemble changes seen in the vaginal epithelium. Only if

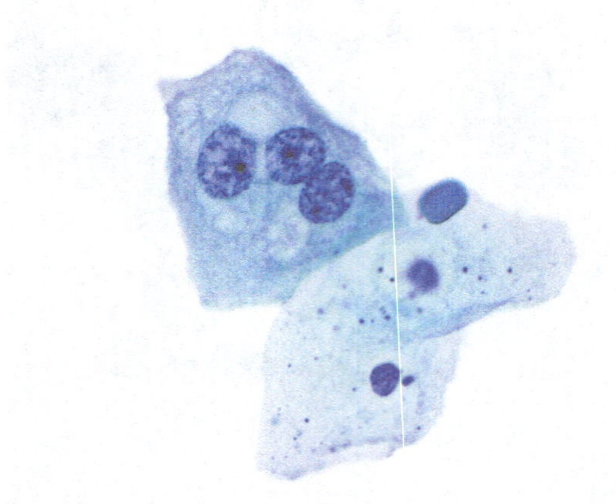

Fig. 3.4 Benign squamous cells. Two benign squamous cells line up below an umbrella cell with three nuclei. The presence of squamous cells in voided urine may come from external genitalia, including the vagina. In a catheterized patient, their origin is usually in an area of metaplasia in the lining of the bladder between the ureteral orifices and the urethra, the trigone (*VU, TP, medium mag.*)

there are tangible abnormal nuclear changes in the squamous cells should the sample be placed into the atypical category. In younger women it can indicate contamination from the cervix or vagina but, in an older population, it may point to an underlying HGUC with squamous differentiation.

Glandular Cells

In voided urine from women, benign glandular cells (Fig. 3.5a, b) may be derived from the uterine cervix or corpus and are usually few and degenerated. Endometrial cells may appear in voided urine specimens in women of all ages. Endometrial-type cells are characterized as cohesive, three-dimensional aggregates of small glandular cells with scant cytoplasm, slightly irregular nuclei with vesicular fine chromatin, and visible small nucleoli. A few clusters in a menstruating woman are of no consequence. However, when the patient is menopausal, and endometrial cells in her voided urine are present, this is an alert to her clinicians (see Chap. 8).

In urine collected by bladder instrumentation, glandular type cells from the urinary tract will be well preserved, with small nuclei and vacuolated cytoplasm. Most often they are true tissue fragments, but also can be seen as single cells. Their origins are many: glandular epithelium in the dome of the bladder (urachal remnant) or trigone are developmental, not metaplasias. Endometriosis may involve the urinary tract, and present an unexpected cellular picture of very small hyperchromatic cells, either in voided urine or brushings from the ureter (see Fig. 3.5a); cells from Mullerian rests (Mullerianosis) are also native, albeit rare (see Fig. 3.5b). Conversely,

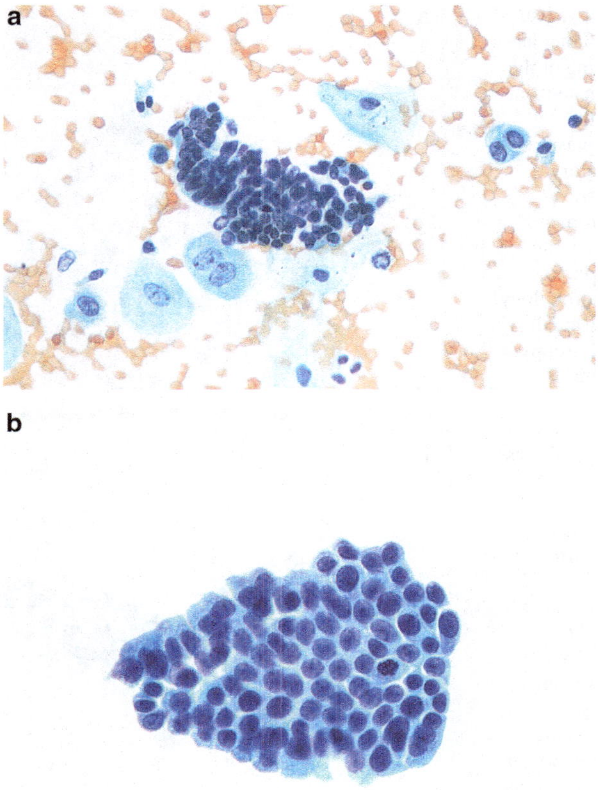

Fig. 3.5 Benign glandular cells—endometriosis, Mullerianosis. (**a**) Glandular cells in a urinary tract specimen may be native to the urinary collecting system, or external to it. The larger cells are urothelial or squamous. The cluster of small dark cells originated in an endometriosis of the ureter. The patient was presenting with hematuria and pain coincident with the patient's menstrual periods (*Ureteral brushing, CS, high mag.*). (**b**) Glandular cells from a focus of Mullerianosis are not distinguishable from other glandular cells in the urinary bladder. This very rare lesion is related to endometriosis, both considered a metaplasia. Their origin must be biopsy proven correlating the morphology with the location deep in the bladder wall (*Bladder washing, SP, medium mag.*)

cystitis cystica/glandularis (Fig. 3.6a–c) is a metaplasia of the urothelium resulting from chronic inflammation.

Renal tubular epithelial cells (Fig. 3.7 a–c) will usually appear degenerated and resemble histiocytes (see Fig. 3.7a), especially if single. Those from the proximal and distal convoluted tubules may appear quite columnar, especially in a true tissue fragment (see Fig. 3.7b) or a cast, whereas those from the loop of Henle will still look like histiocytes, even when seen as an intact cast (see Fig. 3.7c).

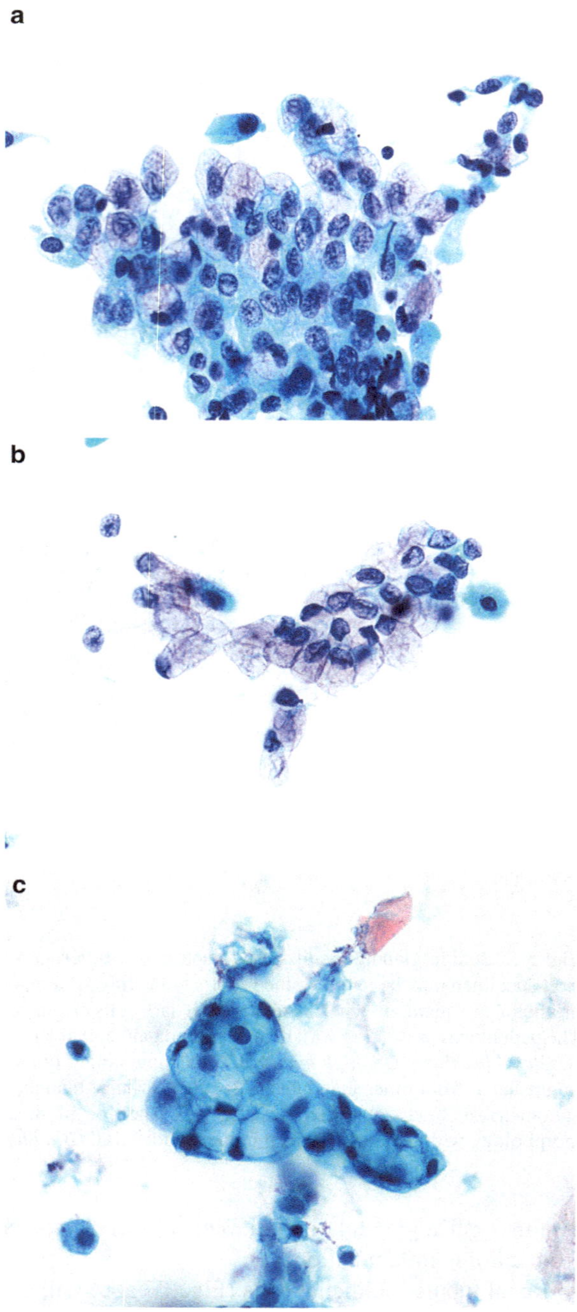

Fig. 3.6 Cystitis cystica/glandularis. (**a**) Glandular cells from the lining of the bladder can originate from a focus native to the urothelium, metaplasia from an inflammatory focus (cystitis cystica/glandularis), or from a glandular neoplasm either primary or secondary. Unless the cytomorphology suggests a neoplasm, all such TTFs or cell groups are considered benign (*Washing, TP, high mag.*). (**b**) Cystitis cystica may appear as in Fig. 3.6a or as a single layer of glandular cells. They closely resemble endocervical cells, and could be from a case of endocervicosis if the tumor was also in the muscular wall of the bladder or ureter. This mucosal strip was from a focus of cystitis cystica (*Washing, TP, high mag.*). (**c**) Another tight glandular group, a TTF, demonstrates nuclear compression by relatively large cytoplasmic vacuoles. Regardless of their origin, these cells fulfill the criteria of benignity, making the diagnosis of "Negative" appropriate (*Washing, TP, high mag.*)

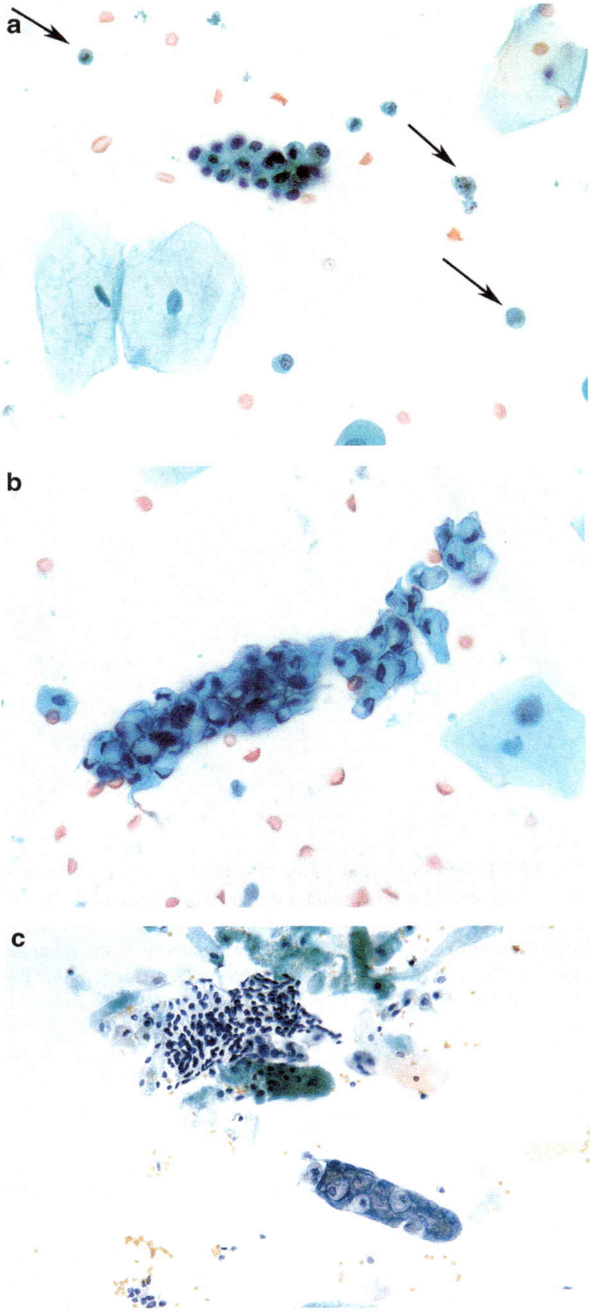

Fig. 3.7 Renal tubular epithelial cells (RTEC). (**a**) RTEC—histiocytic type: RTEC can be very small, the size of histiocytes. They may have vacuolated cytoplasm in varying amounts and may occur singly (*arrows*) in urinary samples. When aggregated as this group, a cast should be considered, implying renal disease. There are usually variable amounts of cellular degeneration (*Voided, SP, high mag.*). (**b**) RTEC—glandular. This large TTF of RTEC is unusual in size, and represents a tubular cast. The renal tubular cells vary from small with scant cytoplasm to larger and vacuolated. The patient was in renal failure (*Voided, SP, high mag.*). (**c**) RTEC—cast. RTEC within this cast demonstrate small nuclei with relatively abundant cytoplasm. The material supporting the RTEC in the cast is protein. The patient was in renal failure (*Voided, CS, high mag.*)

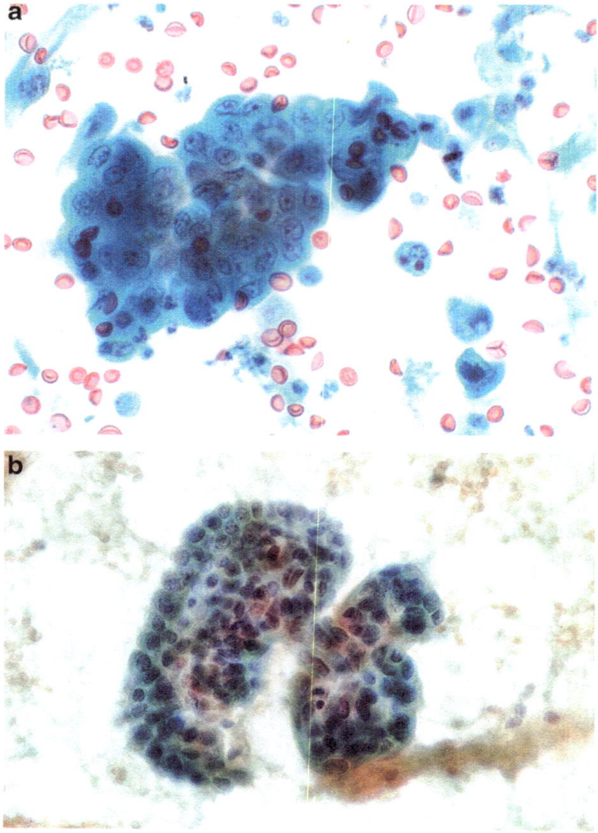

Fig. 3.8 Benign urothelial tissue fragment (BUTF). (**a**) Voided. BUTF can be seen in voided urines, and should not mandate a diagnosis of "atypical". In this fragment, nuclei are uniform in size and shape, evenly spaced, and with finely granular chromatin (*Voided, SP, high mag.*). (**b**) Instrumented from renal pelvis. Cell fragments from the renal pelvis should be cautiously considered. In this case, the diagnosis rendered was "suspicious for low-grade neoplasm". The excision of the kidney revealed only urothelial hyperplasia overlying a subepithelial hemangioma. Retrospective review recognized the uniform nuclear size and round shape. The resemblance to a papillary lesion was no doubt the result of instrumentation (*Renal pelvic washing, CS, high mag.*)

Benign Urothelial Tissue Fragments

Benign Urothelial Tissue Fragments in Voided Urine

Although most cytologists regard urothelial tissue fragments in voided urines (UTF) as abnormal, a recent review of such samples has found them commonplace and benign [11]. Causes of BUTF (Fig. 3.8a) in voided urines are multifold, and include: prostate/rectal manipulation prior to collection of the sample, jogging, abdominal palpation, etc. Most often BUTF are of no clinical importance. Table 3.1 demonstrates

Table 3.1 Significance of benign urothelial tissue fragments (BUTF) and atypical urothelial tissue fragments (AUTF) in voided urines [11, 12]

Follow-up diagnosis	No. (%) BUTF	No. (%) AUTF
Histopathology	29 (10.6)	24 (14.1)
Benign	17 (6.2)	6 (3.5)
Urothelial neoplasia	12 (4.4)	17 (10.0)
PUNLMP	1 (0.4)	0 (0.0)
LGUC	9 (3.3)	2 (1.2)
HGUC	2 (0.7)	15 (8.8)
Cytopathology	45 (16.4)	25 (14.7)
Benign/AUC		
Urolithiasis (Clinical/radiologic/gross)	45 (16.4)	49 (28.8)
No follow-up	25 (9.1)	10 (5.9)

the results of slide review of cases that contained BUTF and atypical urothelial tissue fragments (AUTF) with their follow-up. The results are impressive, and support the fact that cytomorphology and architecture are the most important criteria to suspect LGUN [12] when interpreting the sample; however, the presence of AUTF is more commonly present in tissue-confirmed LGUC than BUTF.

Benign Urothelial Tissue Fragments in Instrumented Urine

Instrumented urine specimens are often cellular, consisting of numerous benign-appearing cells arranged in groups that resemble papillary clusters with smooth (community) borders, and that lack fibrovascular cores (Fig. 3.8b). These are defined as "true tissue fragments" and need to be considered by the cytologist as to their category placement. This will depend upon their nuclear and architectural details. If all the criteria of benign urothelial cells, as outlined above, are present then the call is BUTF and the sample is considered NHGUC, unless other criteria of atypia, suspicious or HGUC are present in the specimen, or if evidence of another significant lesion, e.g., LGUN, is seen [13].

The causes of such BUTF may be neoplasm, recent or concurrent instrumentation, or most commonly, lithiasis of the urinary tract, usually in the renal pelvis (See discussion under section "Risk of Malignancy").

Clusters, Groups, or Sheets of Urothelial Cells

Clusters/groups or sheets of benign urothelial cells (Fig. 3.9a,b), visually different from BUTF (see Fig. 3.8), are commonly found in benign samples and have no significance, so long as the nuclei bear benign characteristics.

Explanatory Note: Instrumented urine specimens include any specimen that was obtained by any instrument or whenever force was applied to dislodge individual cells from the lining urothelium. These include catheterized urines, bladder washings,

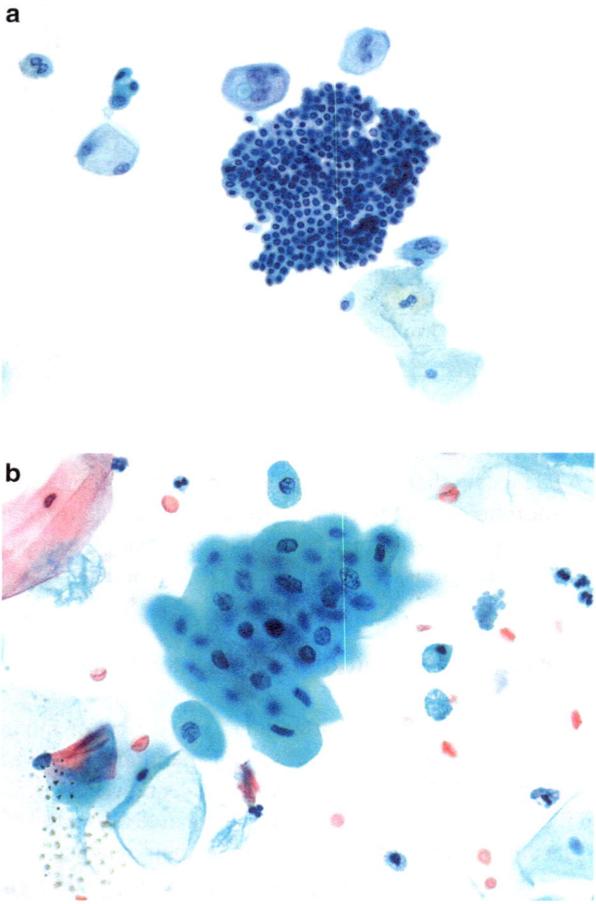

Fig. 3.9 Clusters or sheets of urothelial cells. (**a**) If sheets or clusters have "windows" they cannot be considered TTFs, BUTFs, or AUTFs if they have no atypia. This sheet is essentially a monolayer of uniform cells with round nuclei and uniformly pale chromatin. N/C ratios are high, a reflection of the intermediate position of these cells in the urothelial layer (*Washing, TP, medium mag.*). (**b**) Urothelial cells may undergo squamous metaplasia, indicated by their opaque cytoplasm and sharp cellular borders. Nuclei are small. All of these features indicate a cell group that may be a BUTF, and is certainly benign (*Voided, SP, high mag.*)

brushings, and upper urinary tract urine specimens obtained by urinary catheterization. In addition, any immediately post-cystoscopy urine specimen is also considered instrumented. In general, these specimens are cellular, and the presence of BUTF in instrumented urine specimens is a normal finding; therefore, we should avoid the term "atypia" in this context in these types of specimens so long as the nuclear and architectural features of the UTF do not warrant another diagnosis.

Three-Dimensional Urothelial Tissue Fragments with Nephrolithiasis

Voided urine specimens from patients who may present with hematuria and/or filling defect on imaging studies are often cellular and consist of three-dimensional urothelial fragments composed of cells that may exhibit significant pleomorphism (Fig. 3.10a, b). These three-dimensional urothelial fragments display smooth (community) borders, and cytoplasmic collars/collarets, i.e., a rim of cytoplasm surrounding the nuclei as in BUTF. If a cause of the atypia is found, such as a stone (Fig. 3.10c), then the diagnostic category should be NHGUC.

Urothelium with Nephrolithiasis: Sheets or Clusters/Groups

There may also be sheets or clusters of cells that are not true tissue fragments (see Fig. 3.8a, b). The cells in the fragments or clusters may also exhibit nuclear enlargement and atypia, slightly increased N/C ratios, nuclear and cytoplasmic degeneration, and/or squamous metaplasia (Fig. 3.11a). With a confident diagnosis of lithiasis, and without single HGUC cells in the sample, the findings may be placed in the NHGUC category. If there are any truly atypical well-preserved single cells (Fig. 3.11b), the sample needs to be considered either AUC or Suspicious for HGUC (SHGUC) based upon the criteria for those categories. Occasionally, crystalline material from the stone will support the diagnosis (Fig. 3.11c).

Explanatory Note: Urolithiasis, first noted as a cause of false-positive diagnoses by Papanicolaou, continues to be one of the most significant pitfalls in urinary cytopathology. The clinical history is crucial to avoid a false-positive diagnosis. As described above, BUTF may be seen in instrumented urines and sometimes in voided urine from patients with stones. In general, presence of BUTF in voided urine warrants consideration as they may raise suspicion of an LGUN; however, this diagnosis has to be made based upon the criteria described in Chap. 7. Urothelial carcinoma and squamous cell carcinoma have been associated with renal calculi or infection. The incidence of coexisting urinary stone disease with squamous carcinoma varied from 18 % in US to 100 % in Hong Kong [14, 15] during the 1980s. Two more recent papers [16, 17] support the commonly held belief that staghorn calculi can occur coincidentally with renal pelvic neoplasms. Whether there is a true causal relationship is not clear. However, in the most recent experience, patients with renal pelvic stones present more often with BUTF or AUTF, not with neoplasms [11, 12]. The reasons for these variable experiences are not apparent.

Urothelial Changes Characteristic of Infectious Processes

Acute Bacterial Infections

In the urinary bladder these infections may cause generalized reactive changes in the urothelium that have been discussed above (see Fig. 3.3). Urine specimens from acute bacterial infections are sometimes cellular, consisting of reactive urothelial

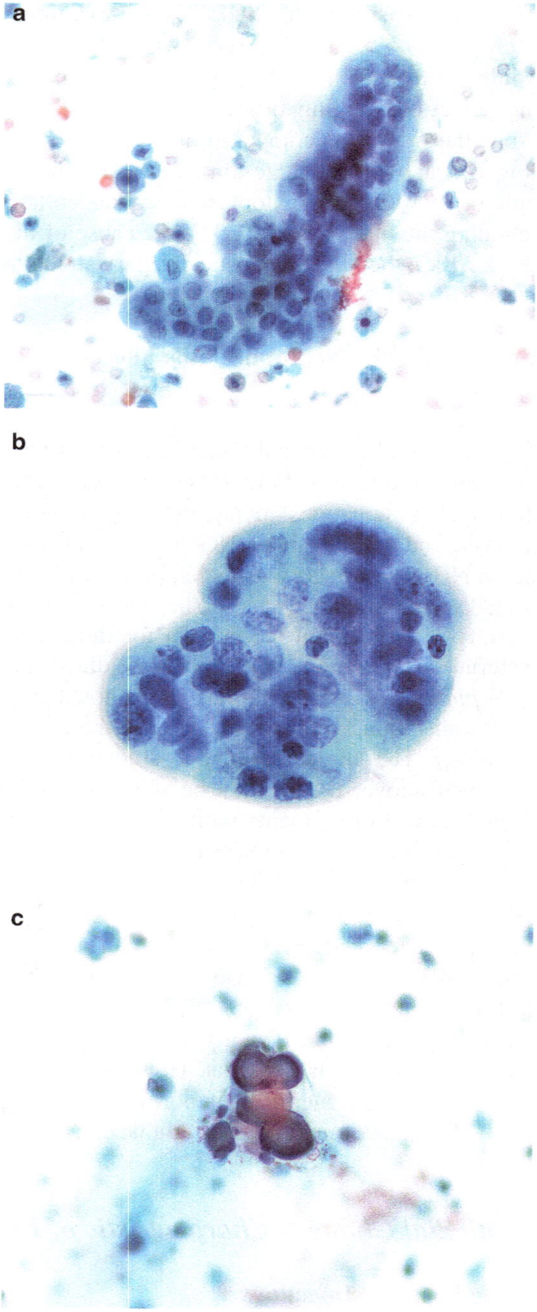

Fig. 3.10 Urothelium with nephrolithiasis—three-dimensional fragments. (**a**) Kidney and bladder stones can cause serious changes in the urothelium, sometimes resembling neoplasms. Careful examination of the cells in a three-dimensional TTF is critical to an accurate diagnosis. These cells have round nuclei which are evenly spaced. Chromatin is finely granular and nucleoli are inconspicuous. A renal calculus was discovered on imaging studies and from the clinical history (*Voided, SP, moderate mag.*). (**b**) A BUTF in a voided urine may be the result of numerous causes. In this patient, nephrolithiasis was the reason. Cellular changes are mild when compared to those in the photos to follow (Chap. 4). The absence of any fibrovascular stalk eliminates the diagnosis of a low grade LGUN (*Voided, SP, high mag.*). (**c**) Calcific concretions in voided urine may be recovered in patients with history of renal calculi (*Voided, SP, high mag.*)

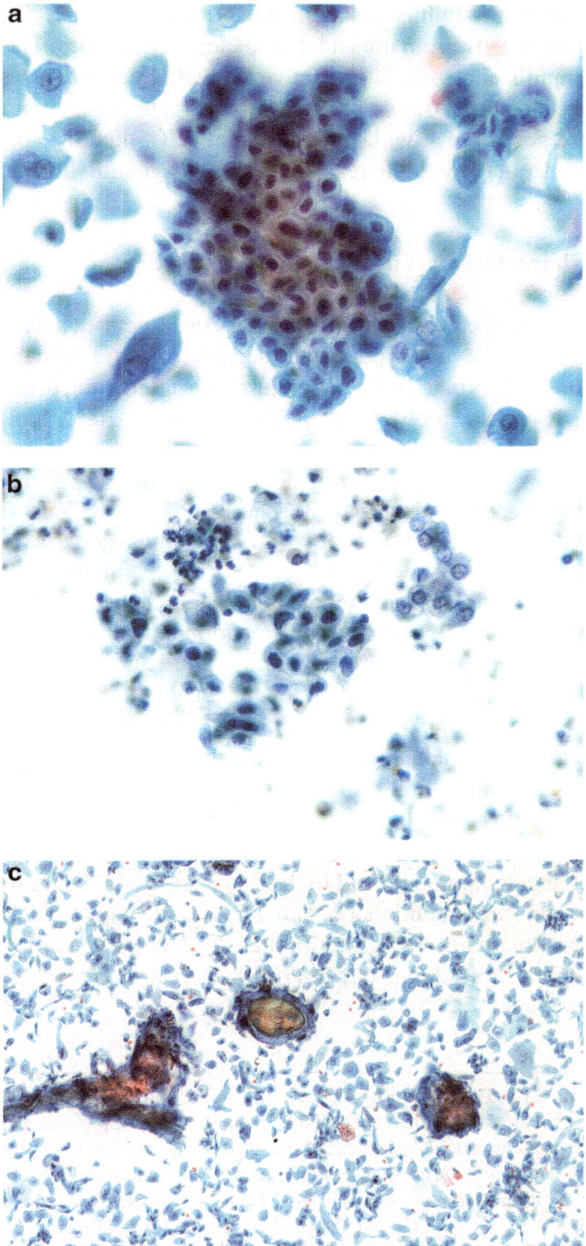

Fig. 3.11 Urothelium with nephrolithiasis—sheets or clusters. (**a**) A sheet of urothelium consists of relatively uniform cells with moderately hyperchromatic nuclei. Even though the nuclear chromatin is darker than normal, the presence of a bladder stone is reason enough for the changes. Because of the history and mild changes, this sample was placed in the "Negative" category (*Voided, SP, moderate mag.*). (**b**) Compare the cells in the center of the field with those to the right, especially considering the nuclear chromatin and nuclear shapes. The central cells are hyperchromatic and the shapes vary. Inflammation is seen in the background. Without the history of nephrolithiasis, these cells would indicate a diagnosis of "atypical urothelial cells" (AUC). If there were any consideration of a urothelial lesion in addition to lithiasis, a note is appropriate or a diagnosis of AUC (*Washing, CS, moderate mag.*). (**c**) Most often direct evidence of stones is not so dramatic as in this photograph. Variation in cells in the background can be appreciated (*Washing, SP, low mag.*)

cells with slightly enlarged nuclei and prominent nucleoli, but with fine, evenly distributed chromatin and thin nuclear membranes. The presence of infiltrating neutrophils admixed with reactive urothelial cells supports a reactive, benign process (acute cystitis), as do clusters of bacteria in the background. If the predominant cells are neutrophils, with rare urothelial cells, then the specimen should be considered inadequate, with the reason for that designation included in the report.

Characteristic Viral Cytopathic Effects

In urine specimens these characteristic effects include Herpes simplex virus, usually type II, but also type I; cytomegalovirus: and human papillomavirus (HPV). The most important and most common virus identified in urine specimens is polyoma (BK or very rarely JC) virus (Fig. 3.12a–e). Human polyoma viruses are small, non-enveloped double-stranded DNA viruses that are classified into two main strains that may infect the urinary tract, named after the initials of the patients from whom they were first identified (BK and JC) [18]. Polyoma virus infected cells are enlarged with single, homogeneous basophilic inclusions occupying most of the enlarged nuclear area (see Fig. 3.12a). Nuclear membranes of those cells are smooth and regular in shape as compared to the irregular nuclear membranes in high-grade malignant cells, which they often mimic (decoy cells). When these cells degenerate, the basophilia clears as the chromatin extrudes, leaving a spider web of residual chromatin. Usually, only a few infected cells are found (see Fig. 3.12b, c).

Explanatory Note 1: In cytology samples, numerous neutrophils admixed with reactive urothelial cells often containing prominent nucleoli indicate a reactive process. These findings, in an appropriate clinical setting, should not trigger the diagnosis of atypia in these specimens, but should place them in the NHGUC category.

Explanatory Note 2: Similarly, the presence of cells with well-recognized viral changes should not lead to the diagnosis of AUC. Primary polyoma virus infections occur during childhood and are usually subclinical. Over 90 % of adults are seropositive for viral antibodies. The virus generally remains latent in the renal tubular epithelium but intermittent viruria can be detected in 0.3 % of healthy

Fig. 3.12 Polyoma virus—classic (**a**), spider web (**b**)–(**c**), benign case (**d**)–(**e**). (**a**) Polyoma cytopathic effect is often seen in patients with immunosuppression from a variety of causes. The classic changes include enlargement of the nucleus and nuclear chromatin homogenization, caused by the viral infection. The shape of the nucleus is always round or oval with a very smooth outline. Cytoplasm is almost gone (*Voided, SP, high mag.*). (**b**) In addition to the classic changes described in Fig. 3.12a, dissolution of the nuclear chromatin is also a characteristic of polyoma (BK) virus infection. The size and shape of the nucleus are the same as the classic features (*Voided, SP, high mag.*). (**c**) If the focal plane is changed, then a spider web of degenerated chromatin comes into view (*Voided, SP, high mag.*). (**d**) The assortment of pale and darker cells is striking on low magnification (Washing, *TP, low mag.*). (**e**) Closer view will demonstrate the reasons for the dark cells observed on low magnification (Fig. 3.12d). Almost all the cells display glassy nuclear inclusions diagnostic of Polyoma virus (*Washing, TP, high mag.*)

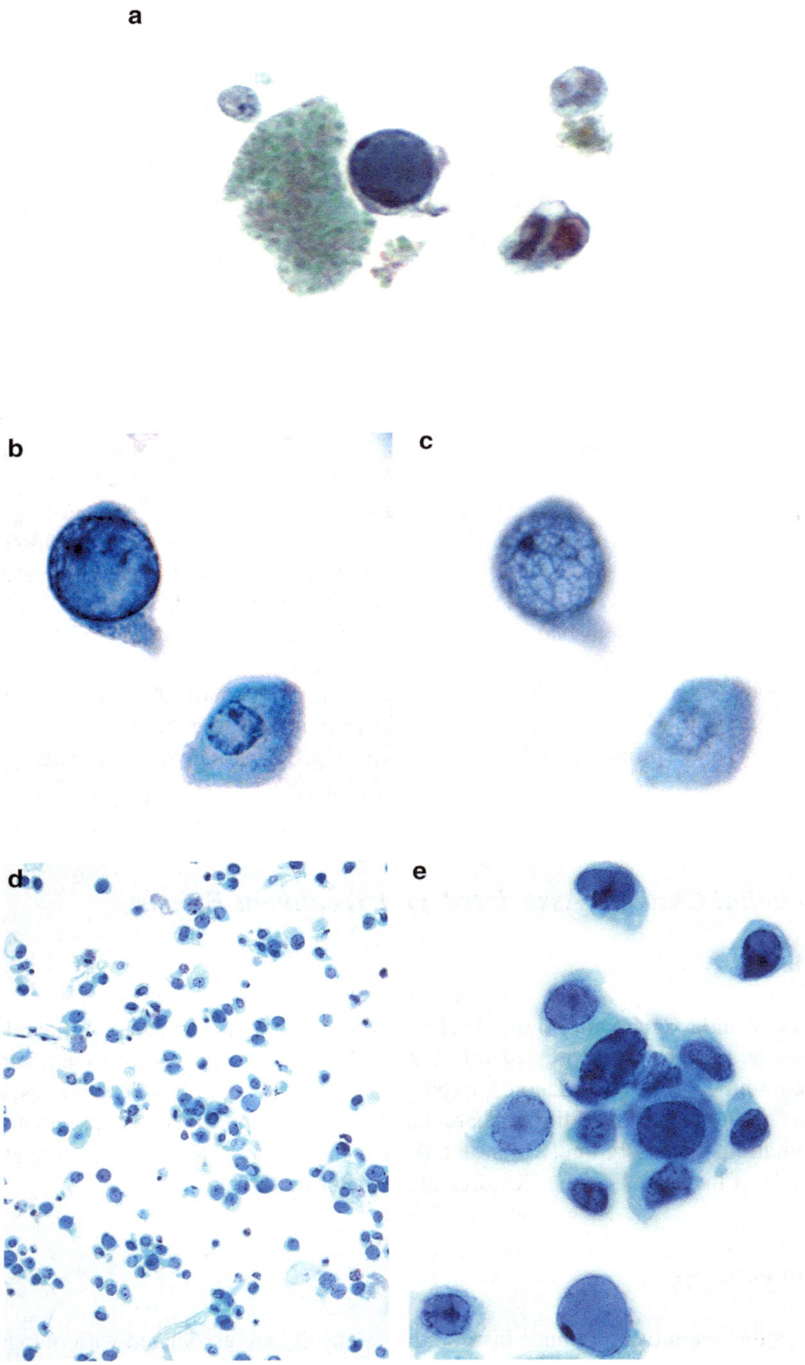
a
b
c
d
e

adults. The infection is reactivated in individuals with various degrees of immunological deficit. In renal transplant recipients, polyoma virus nephropathy occurs in 3–5 % of patients and loss of transplant occurs in 50 % of those affected [18]. Once polyoma virus is detected, immunosuppression has to be lowered.

Explanatory note 3: The infected cells can easily be misclassified as malignant. Therefore, they were referred to as “decoy cells”, analogous to “decoy ducks” used in hunting wild ducks, by Andrew Ricci [19], a cytotechnologist working in the cytology laboratory of Memorial Sloan Kettering Cancer Center, and popularized by Leopold Koss in the second edition of his influential textbook, *Diagnostic Cytology and Its Histopathologic Bases* [20, 21]. In addition, urothelial cells infected by polyoma virus have an abnormal DNA count and can be a potential pitfall for any DNA-based tests, including FISH [21–24]. Once cellular changes are attributed to a polyoma virus infection, those specimens should not be called atypical. However, polyoma virus can infect malignant cells, so if a cell has features of polyoma virus but an irregular nuclear shape, careful search of the specimen is warranted to find diagnostic cells of malignancy if present (see Fig. 3.12.d, e).

Explanatory Note 4: VandenBussche and colleagues, in a recent and as yet unpublished study, found that of 107 cases reviewed, 67 (63 %) were reclassified from AUC to benign. During evaluation, the two reviewers disagreed on the reclassification of 40 (37 %) cases and a third pathologist served as adjudicator. 27 (46 %) cases with disagreement had degenerative changes, compared to 31 (53 %) cases with agreement ($p=0.58$). 34 (51 %) cases that were reclassified as benign had degenerative changes, compared to 24 (60 %) cases that remained classified as AUC ($p=0.42$). None of the contentious cases had sufficient differences to be considered significant, underlining the difficulty in classifying BK viral changes into benign or atypical.

Urothelial Changes Associated with Treatment Effects

Radiation

Radiation-induced cytomorphologic changes will display significant cytomegaly and nucleomegaly, and a preserved N/C ratio. Multinucleation may be seen, and nuclear and cytoplasmic vacuoles, larger than the native cytoplasmic vacuoles, are often demonstrated. In addition, characteristic polychromasia can be appreciated. Chromatin is generally finely granular. All of these changes place the sample as NHGUC if there are no other features of atypia or malignancy.

Immunotherapy

Certain therapeutic compounds instilled intravesically are associated with recognizable changes in urine specimens. Intravesical BCG immunotherapy can cause granulomatous inflammation in urine specimens (Fig. 3.13a, b). In post-BCG cytology

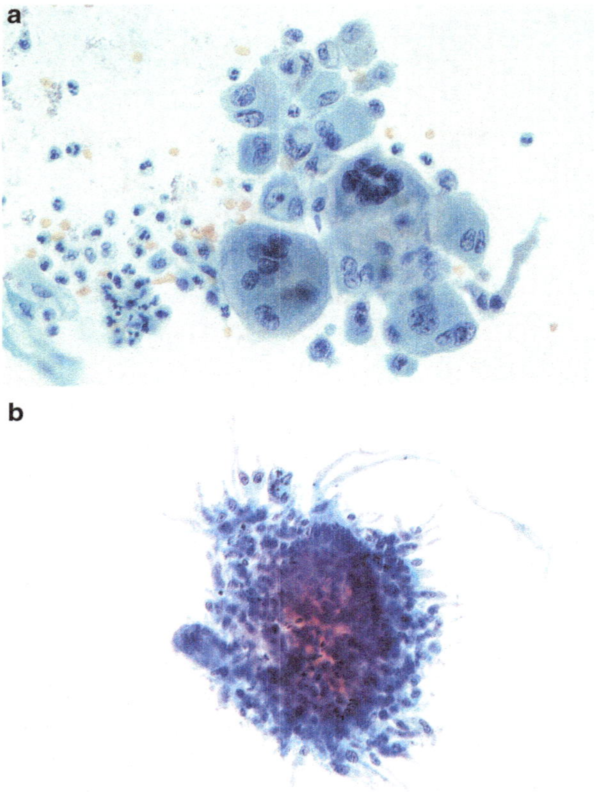

Fig. 3.13 Granulomatous reaction following BCG immunotherapy. (**a**) Multinucleation in usual superficial cells is common. In contrast, Langhans-type giant cells resulting from fused macrophages are multinucleated but have their smaller and slightly hyperchromatic nuclei clustered at one pole of the cytoplasm. Clinical history revealed recent BCG instillation following diagnosis of bladder cancer (*Voided, CS, high mag.*). (**b**) In addition to Langhans giant cells, granulomas can be found in urines following BCG immunotherapy. These granulomas are no different from any other body site, complete with monocytes, lymphocytes, and histiocytes in a tight mélange (*Washing, TP, high mag.*)

urine specimens, granulomas are composed of epithelioid histiocytes admixed with lymphocytes. Occasionally, multinucleated histiocytic giant cells are also seen. Once again, the presence of granulomas in an appropriate clinical setting, i.e., in patients treated with BCG, should not trigger the diagnosis of atypia in urine specimens.

Chemotherapy

On the other hand, intravesical mitomycin and thiotepa usually affect superficial cells and cause nuclear enlargement, multinucleation and hyperchromasia of those cells, all of which are non-specific but may be worrisome. Systemic cyclophosphamide

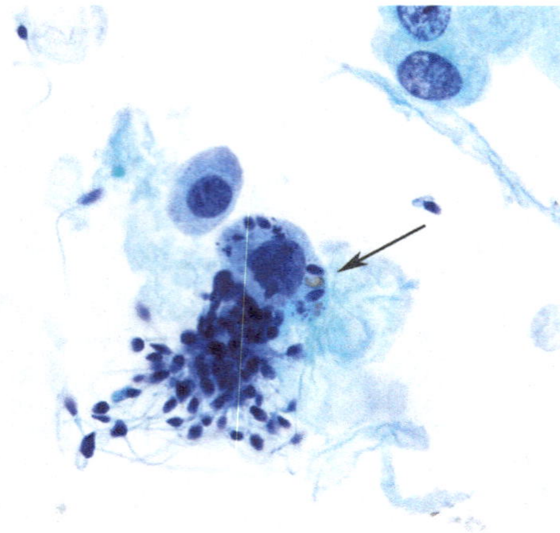

Fig. 3.14 Seminal vesicle cells are unusual, and may provide confusion with HGUC cells because of their large size and nuclear hyperchromasia. Two clues to their identity include intracytoplasmic yellow lipofuscin pigment (*arrow*), and accompanying sperm (*Washing, TP, high mag.*)

(Cytoxan), given for reasons other than urothelial malignancy, has been reported to be associated with urothelial hyperchromasia and degeneration, plus the presence of large nuclei and increased N/C ratios. Ancillary testing, such as FISH, can be very helpful in such instances. Refer to Chap. 9, for further discussion of clinical/prognostic implications of FISH results.

Seminal Vesicle Cells

Sporadically occurring and scarce, degenerated seminal vesicle cells (Fig. 3.14) can be seen in urine specimens, particularly from older patients, especially after a digital rectal examination or prostatic massage.

Seminal vesicle cells in urine specimens often have a bizarre appearance with greatly enlarged nuclei and foamy fragmented minimal cytoplasm. The chromatin is hyperchromatic, degenerated, and smudgy. In contrast, the chromatin of malignant cells is coarse. As in prostatic specimens, seminal vesicle cells may be distinguished from cancer cells by the presence of golden brown lipofuscin pigment. Often mature spermatozoa accompany seminal vesicle cells.

Explanatory Note: Seminal vesicle cells have an abnormal DNA content and potentially are a pitfall for DNA-based adjuvant tests. When seminal vesicle cells are recognized by the presence of yellow pigment and mature spermatozoa in the background, there is no need to call the urine specimen atypical.

Bladder Diversion Urine

Urinary diversion specimens are urines obtained from patients who underwent cystectomy and one of the surgical procedures designed to reroute the urine flow (ileal conduit, Indiana pouch, or neobladder). All of these procedures use a portion of small bowel (ileum) that is anastomosed to the ureters and/or urethra.

Urine specimens are very cellular and composed mainly of degenerated glandular cells, either single or in clusters, resembling dying histiocytes, in a dirty background with mucus and bacteria (Fig. 3.15a). Well-preserved enteric glandular cells may be seen in samples from newly constructed diversion pouches (Fig. 3.15b). Often urothelial cells from upper tracts are present and may show marked degeneration. Characteristics of degeneration are large red intracytoplasmic inclusions, so-called Melamed–Wolinska bodies, which are often seen in these cells (Fig. 3.16). Careful search for HGUC is the primary role of the cytologist (Fig. 3.17a, b).

Explanatory Note: The purpose of cytologic evaluation of urinary diversion specimens is to monitor the upper tract in patients with a history of urothelial carcinoma. For all practical purposes, all of these specimens appear "atypical" due to marked degeneration. The diagnosis of malignancy should be made only if clear criteria of malignancy, usually HGUC, have been met. Otherwise these specimens should be categorized as NHGUC. Rarely, patients will develop adenocarcinoma in their diversion "bladder"; cytologic changes are consistent with gastrointestinal adenocarcinomas [25].

The Rate of Negative Samples in a Usual Laboratory Population

The rate of each diagnostic category depends upon the population served by the laboratory. Referral centers, with oncologic urologists, will undoubtedly have much larger rates of "Suspicious for" (SHGUC) and outright HGUC than reference laboratories serving general practitioners and internists. Having established a baseline figure for each category, every laboratory is wise to watch for "diagnostic drift", wherein the indeterminate categories become wastebaskets, influencing the rate of the adjacent categories; in urinary cytology, AUC can catch the overflow of difficult cases from the NHGUC and SHGUC categories. Careful cytohistologic correlation with microscopic review of challenging cases by all concerned, i.e., cytotechnologists and cytopathologists together, will achieve an even playing field of diagnoses, so important to clinical management. Direct communication with clinicians, especially in suspected lesions of the upper urinary tract, is essential to patient safety.

From an informal survey for The Paris System, the percentage of diagnostic categories in academic and private practice laboratories has been gathered (Table 3.2). The large range of the category of AUC is the most troubling one, as it provides no useful information to the urologist or healthcare provider seeing the patient.

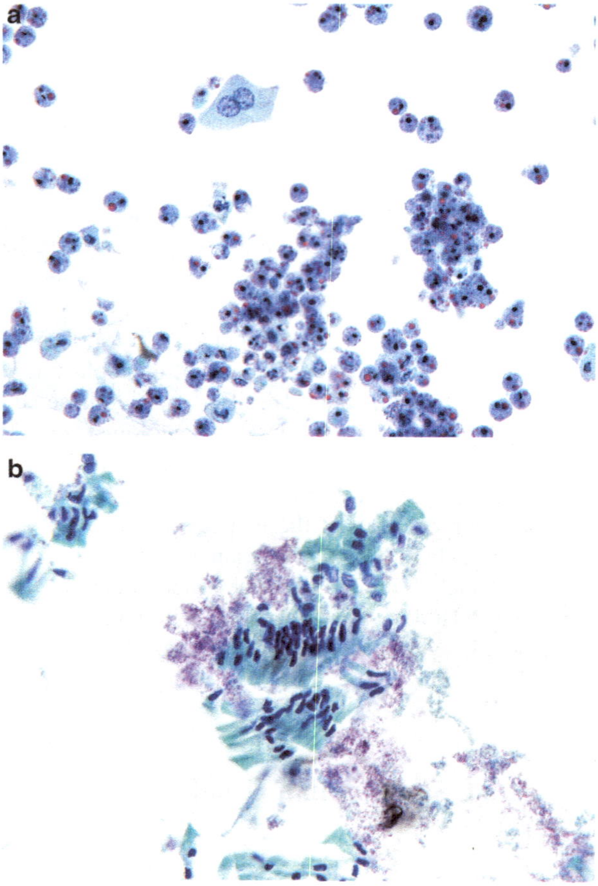

Fig. 3.15 Enteric cells following a urinary diversion post-cystectomy. (**a**) One superficial urothelial cell is present to conveniently compare with the small round cells in the figure. All are of the same size and have small punctate nuclei. These are typical of degenerated enteric cells (*Catheterized, TP, medium mag.*). (**b**) Following a cystectomy, a diversionary pouch is constructed, lined by cells from the portion of the intestine used. Remarkably, the cells don't undergo metaplasia because of the toxic urine, but they do degenerate. They usually are single and closely resemble histiocytes. Sometimes they cluster, which can present a diagnostic dilemma. Careful focusing will reveal the small nuclei, dissimilar to HGUC (*Catheterized, SP, medium mag.*)

The stricter the criteria for that category, and the less often it is used, the more meaningful the cytologic method is to our urologic patients. Most of those samples will doubtless fit best in the NHGUC category when the criteria are observed. Atypia should not be used just because the cells do not quite look normal. Since The Paris System is designed to convey risk, the AUC category must have some meaning.

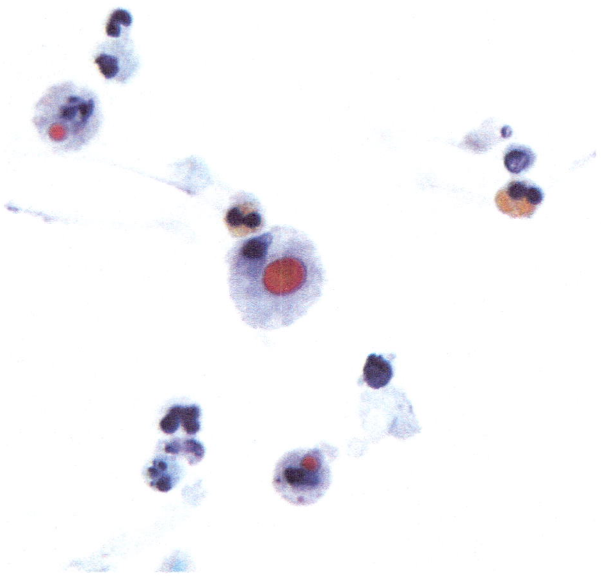

Fig. 3.16 Melamed–Wolinska bodies. Characteristic of degeneration, these intracytoplasmic *round red* inclusions have stymied cytologists for years. No one has ever identified their chemical properties, but they are definitely a benign change, unassociated with malignancy (*Voided, TP, high mag.*)

Risk of Malignancy

The published rate of follow-up biopsy after negative or benign urine cytology ranges from 3.4 to 6.2 % with 32.2–68.9 % of the biopsies revealing low/high-grade urothelial carcinoma [1, 26, 27]. Brimo et al. showed that in cytologically benign cases, symptomatic screening and urothelial cancer surveillance detected high-grade urothelial cancer or carcinoma in situ in 16 of 103 (15.5 %) cases at follow-up biopsy [26]. The likelihood ratios associated with benign urine cytology depend on specimen type (voided vs. instrumented) and grade (low or high) of urothelial carcinoma [28] (Table 3.3).

In the literature, the false- negative rate of ileal conduit and neobladder urinary diversion is 5.7–8.7 % [29, 30]. Although usually benign, patients with extensive intestinal metaplasia involving the urinary tract are at risk of developing subsequent bladder adenocarcinoma [31].

Galed-Placed et al. reported a rare case of decoy and malignant cells coexisting, and hence, identification of decoy cells does not exclude the existence of carcinoma [32, 33]. Even the utilization of IHC with SV40 antibody to prove the presence of BK virus does not confirm or disprove that HGUC is also present. In both instances of malignant transformation, the incidence of these situations is too rare to estimate risk.

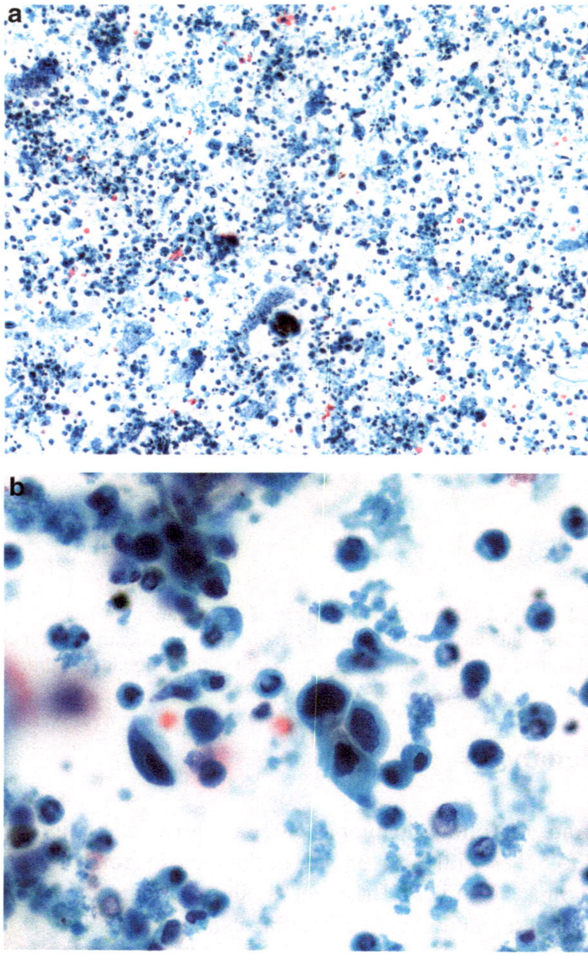

Fig. 3.17 HGUC in a sample of urinary diversion specimen. (**a**) Compare this low magnification view of a highly cellular specimen with Fig. 3.12d. Both scenes are punctuated with dark objects that require closer examination (*Catheterized, SP, low mag.*). (**b**) Higher magnification demonstrates hyperchromatic epithelial cells larger than the surrounding enteric cells. Malignant cells are the goal of examining these specimens: Find the HGUC! (*Catheterized, SP, high mag.*)

Table 3.2 The distribution of diagnostic categories utilized in The Paris System survey in academic and private practice settings (unpublished data)

Total range	Academic	Private practice
Positive (%)	1.0–6.3	1.2–4.9
Suspicious (%)	0.7–5.4	0.2–2.7
Atypical (%)	1.8–23.7	3.1–21.4
Negative (%)	75.4–94.8	71.4–96.1
Washing (%)	1.0–74	1.0–22.2
Number/year	841–9210	81–4932

Table 3.3 The likelihood risk ratios associated with benign urine cytology dependent upon specimen type and grade (low or high) of urothelial carcinoma

Specimen type	Low grade—UC	High grade—UC
Voided	0.738	0.384
Instrumented	0.538	0.162
Upper tract	0.400	0.400

From Raab et al. [28] with kind permission of Springer Science+Business Media

References

1. Rosenthal DL, Vandenbussche CJ, Burroughs FH, Sathiyamoorthy S, Guan H, Owens C. The Johns Hopkins Hospital template for urologic cytology samples: part I-creating the template. Cancer Cytopathol. 2013;121:15–20.
2. Wojcik EM. What should not be reported as atypia in urine cytology. J Am Soc Cytopathol. 2015;4:30–6.
3. Harris MJ, Schwinn CP, Morrow JW, Gray RL, Browell BM. Exfoliative cytology of the urinary bladder irrigation specimen. Acta Cytol. 1971;15:385–99.
4. Hughes JH, Raab SS, Cohen MB. The cytologic diagnosis of low-grade transitional cell carcinoma. Am J Clin Pathol. 2000;114(Suppl):S59–67.
5. Raab SS, Slagel DD, Jensen CS, Teague MW, Savell VH, Ozkutlu D, et al. Low-grade transitional cell carcinoma of the urinary bladder: application of select cytologic criteria to improve diagnostic accuracy [corrected]. Mod Pathol. 1996;9:225–32.
6. Raab SS, Lenel JC, Cohen MB. Low grade transitional cell carcinoma of the bladder. Cytologic diagnosis by key features as identified by logistic regression analysis. Cancer. 1994;74:1621–6.
7. Wojcik EM, Brownlie RJ, Bassler TJ, Miller MC. Superficial urothelial (umbrella) cells. A potential cause of abnormal DNA ploidy results in urine specimens. Anal Quant Cytol Histol. 2000;22:411–5.
8. Zhou AG, Hutchinson LM, Cosar EF. Urine cytopathology and ancillary methods. Surg Pathol Clin. 2014;7:77–88.
9. Reynolds JP, Voss JS, Kipp BR, Karnes RJ, Nassar A, Clayton AC, et al. Comparison of urine cytology and fluorescence in situ hybridization in upper urothelial tract samples. Cancer Cytopathol. 2014;122:459–67.
10. Barkan GA, Wojcik EM. Genitourinary cytopathology (kidney and urinary tract). Cancer Treat Res. 2014;160:149–83.
11. Onur I, Rosenthal DL, VandenBussche CJ. Benign-appearing urothelial tissue fragments in noninstrumented voided urine specimens are associated with low rates of urothelial neoplasia. Cancer Cytopathol. 2015;123:180–5.
12. Onur I, Rosenthal DL, VandenBussche CJ. Atypical urothelial tissue fragments in noninstrumented voided urine specimens are associated with low but significantly higher rates of urothelial neoplasia than benign-appearing urothelial tissue fragments. Cancer Cytopathol. 2015;123:186–92.
13. McCrosky Z, Kliethermes S, Bahar B, Barkan GA, Pambuccian SE, Wojcik E. Is a consistent cytologic diagnosis of low-grade urothelial carcinoma in instrumented urinary tract cytologic specimens possible? J Am Soc Cytopathol. 2015;4:90–7.
14. Blacher EJ, Johnson DE, Abdul-Karmim FW, Ayala AG. Squamous cell carcinoma of the renal pelvis. Urology. 1985;25:124–6.
15. Li MK, Cheung WL. Squamous cell carcinoma of the renal pelvis. J Urol. 1987;138:269–71.
16. Katz R, Gofrit ON, Golijanin D, Landau EH, Shapiro A, Pode D, Meretyk S. Urothelial cancer of the renal pelvis in percutaneous nephrolithotomy patients. Urol Int. 2005;75:17–20.
17. Yeh CC, Lin TH, Wu HC, Chang CH, Chen CC, Chen WC. A high association of upper urinary tract transitional cell carcinoma with nonfunctioning kidney caused by stone disease in Taiwan. Urol Int. 2007;79:19–23.

18. Pinto M, Dobson S. BK and JC virus: a review. J Infect. 2014;68 Suppl 1:S2–8.
19. Paquette C, Elhosseiny A. Significance of polyomavirus detection in urine cytology: an update. Diagn Histopathol. 2012;18:321–6.
20. Koss LG. On decoy cells. Acta Cytol. 2005;49:233–4.
21. Koss LG. Diagnostic cytology and its histopathologic bases. 2nd ed. Philadelphia: J. B. Lippincott; 1968. p. 653.
22. Wojcik EM, Miller MC, Wright BC, Veltri RW, O'Dowd GJ. Comparative analysis of DNA content in polyomavirus-infected urothelial cells, urothelial dysplasia and high grade transitional cell carcinoma. Anal Quant Cytol Histol. 1997;19:430–6.
23. Bakhos R, Shankey TV, Flanigan RC, Fisher S, Wojcik EM. Comparative analysis of DNA flow cytometry and cytology of bladder washings: review of discordant cases. Diagn Cytopathol. 2000;22:65–9.
24. Halling KC, Kipp BR. Bladder cancer detection using FISH (UroVysion assay). Adv Anat Pathol. 2008;15:279–86.
25. Ali-El-Dein B, El-Tabey N, Abdel-Latif M, Abdel-Rahim M, El-Bahnasawy MS. Late uro-ileal cancer after incorporation of ileum into the urinary tract. J Urol. 2002;167:84–8.
26. Brimo F, Vollmer RT, Case B, Aprikian A, Kassouf W, Auger M. Accuracy of urine cytology and the significance of an atypical category. Am J Clin Pathol. 2009;132:785–93.
27. Raab SS, Grzybicki DM, Vrbin CM, Geisinger KR. Urine cytology discrepancies: frequency, causes, and outcomes. Am J Clin Pathol. 2007;127:946–53.
28. Raab SS, Booth CN, Jones JS. Urine cytology. In: Hansel DE, McKenney JK, Stephenson AJ, Chang SS, editors. The urinary tract: a comprehensive guide to patient diagnosis and management. New York: Springer; 2012. p. 293–310.
29. Ajit D, Dighe SB, Desai SB. Cytology of Ileal conduit urine in bladder cancer patients: diagnostic utility and pitfalls. Acta Cytol. 2006;50:70–3.
30. Cimino-Mathews A, Ali SZ. The clinicopathologic correlates of cellular atypia in urinary cytology of ileal neobladders. Acta Cytol. 2011;55:449–54.
31. Koss LG, Hoda RS. Cytologic manifestations of benign disorders affecting cells of the lower urinary tract. In: Koss LG, Hoda RS, editors. Koss's cytology of the urinary tract with histopathology correlations. New York: Springer; 2012. p. 47–71.
32. Galed-Placed I, Valbuena-Ruvira L. Decoy cells and malignant cells coexisting in the urine from a transplant recipient with BK virus nephropathy and bladder adenocarcinoma. Diagn Cytopathol. 2011;39:933–7.
33. Geetha D, Tong BC, Racusen L, Markowitz JS, Westra WH. Bladder carcinoma in a transplant recipient: evidence to implicate the BK human polyomavirus as a causal transforming agent. Transplantation. 2002;73:1933–6.

Chapter 4
Atypical Urothelial Cells (AUC)

Güliz A. Barkan, Tarik M. Elsheikh, Daniel F.I. Kurtycz, Sachiko Minamiguchi, Hiroshi Ohtani, Eric Piaton, Spasenija Savic Prince, Z. Laura Tabatabai, and Christopher J. VandenBussche

Background

Atypical categories are frequently criticized as lacking specificity, reproducibility, and leaving clinicians without a clear course of action; however, they do reflect the real-world possibilities of cytologic diagnoses and inability to place a given case into neatly defined benign and malignant categories. Clinicians may dislike the use of "atypia" and may go as far as to suggest that the use of this term reflects naiveté or incompetence of the pathologist who cannot make a definitive call. Alternatively, the diagnostician may not be able to generate a definitive answer because of lack of well-defined, reliable diagnostic criteria. Historically, the term atypia was introduced to cytopathology by Dr. George N. Papanicolaou, to convey a very low suspicion of malignancy [1].

Today, with the evidence-based approach to morphology, this term fits a real need to fill the gap between what can be recognized as entirely normal and what can be recognized as being clearly abnormal. Laboratory methods cannot always offer discrete cut-off points between diseased and non-diseased states. Therefore, medical science is continually attempting to refine methodologies such that indeterminate categories may be reduced. As eloquently stated by Pambuccian "A clinically meaningful, standardized cytodiagnostic category of 'atypia' requires a distinct definition, quantitative criteria, agreed-upon reference images, a clear clinical meaning (likelihood of underlying malignancy) and, ideally, well-defined management options" [1]. In that spirit, based on the current level of understanding and available evidence, the category of "atypical urothelial cells" (AUC) is offered in the context of The Paris System for Reporting Urinary Cytology.

D.L. Rosenthal et al. (eds.), *The Paris System for Reporting Urinary Cytology*,
DOI 10.1007/978-3-319-22864-8_4

Definition

The general diagnostic category AUC is reserved for specimens that contain urothelial cells with *mild to moderate* cytologic (not architectural) atypia. This definition, therefore, does not include urothelial cell clusters (tissue fragments) without cytologic atypia, which belong in the negative for high-grade urothelial carcinoma category (NHGUC). To be classified as AUC, the cytologic changes have to fall short of a diagnosis of suspicious for high-grade urothelial carcinoma (SHGUC) or high-grade urothelial carcinoma (HGUC) (see Chaps. 5 and 6). In addition, this category requires exclusion of changes in which the reason for "atypia" is known, such as changes caused by polyomavirus and other infections, reactive umbrella cells, seminal vesicle cells, and reactive changes due to stones, instrumentation, and therapy [2]. Such cases should be assigned to the NHGUC category (see Chap. 3). Figures 4.1 and 4.2 depict normal benign/reactive urothelial cells compared to Figs. 4.3, 4.4, 4.5, 4.6, 4.7, 4.8, 4.9, and 4.10, which depict AUC. The AUC category also includes specimens where, due to poor preservation and degenerative changes, the nature and degree of atypia in the urothelial cells cannot be well analyzed. However, it is important to note that the mere presence of degeneration does not warrant the diagnosis of AUC. Degeneration is an expected finding in voided urine samples, especially after delayed processing and in urinary diversion specimens. These changes should not be diagnosed as AUC.

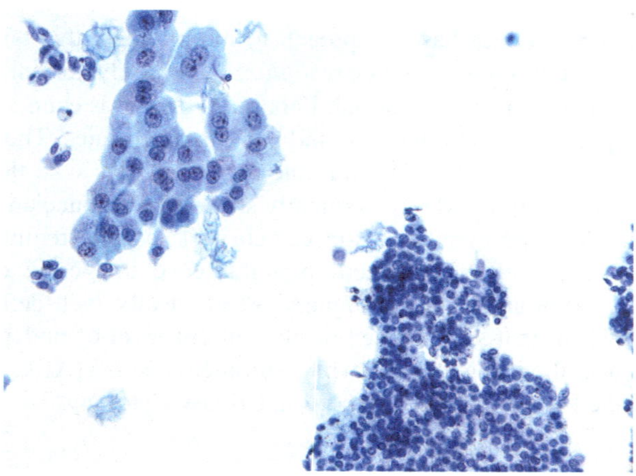

Fig. 4.1 Benign urothelial cells. The *top left corner* shows benign superficial urothelial cells (umbrella cells) and the *bottom right corner* has benign intermediate/basal type urothelial cells. Although the non-superficial urothelial cells have a high N/C ratio, they have a smooth nuclear contour and do not show nuclear enlargement, placing them in the "negative" category. The follow-up diagnosis was benign (*Bladder washing, TP, high mag.*)

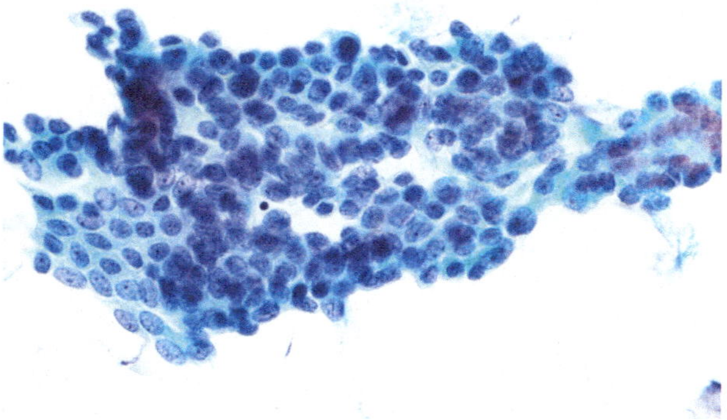

Fig. 4.2 Reactive urothelial cells. Superficial urothelial cells with slight nuclear enlargement and prominent chromocenters. There is no nuclear hyperchromasia, clumped chromatin, or nuclear contour irregularity. These changes are consistent with the "negative" category (*Bladder washing, TP, high mag.*)

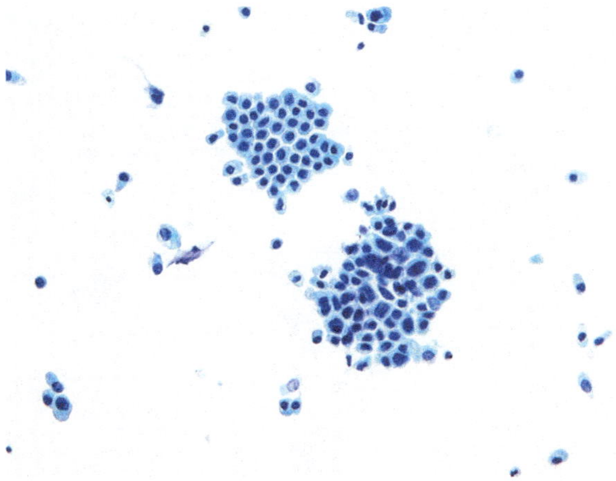

Fig. 4.3 Atypical urothelial cells (AUC). Two groups of urothelial cells are shown. The group at the *top* is composed of intermediate type urothelial cells with smooth nuclear contours, and no features of atypia. The urothelial cells in the group on the *bottom* have high N/C ratios, and nuclear contour irregularity. Nuclear chromasia is similar in both groups. Due to the cytologic atypia seen in the group on the *bottom* this case should be categorized as AUC (*bladder washing, TP, intermediate mag.*)

Criteria

To standardize the criteria of the AUC category, a strict morphological definition based upon the characteristics of AUC is indispensable. The diagnosis AUC is defined as cellular changes that fulfill the major (required) criterion and only one

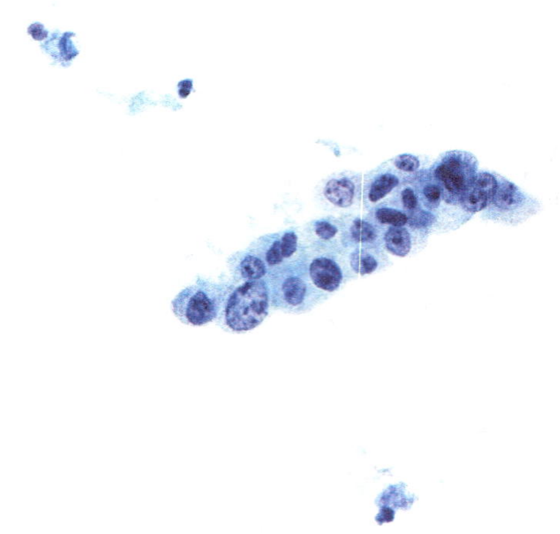

Fig. 4.4 Atypical urothelial cells (AUC). Atypical urothelial cells with high N/C ratios and nuclear contour irregularity. The absence of hyperchromasia and the presence of degenerated clumped chromatin preclude a diagnosis of SHGUC (*Bladder washing, TP, high mag.*)

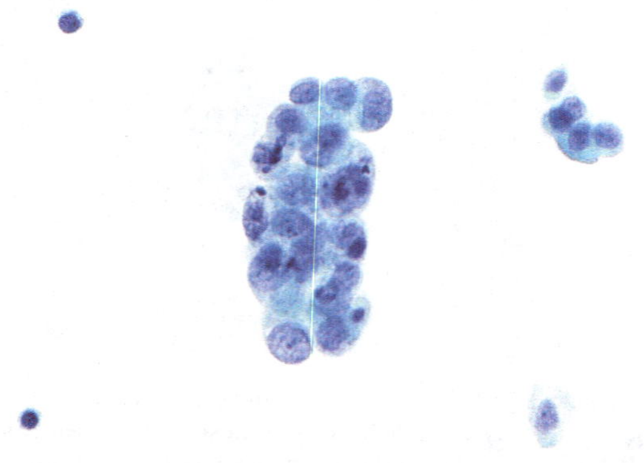

Fig. 4.5 Atypical urothelial cells (AUC). Atypical urothelial cells with high N/C ratio, enlarged nuclei, prominent chromocenters and mild nuclear contour irregularity. The chromatin is unevenly distributed yet hypochromatic. Concurrent bladder biopsy showed acute cystitis with extensive reactive epithelial changes. (*Bladder Washing, TP, high mag.*)

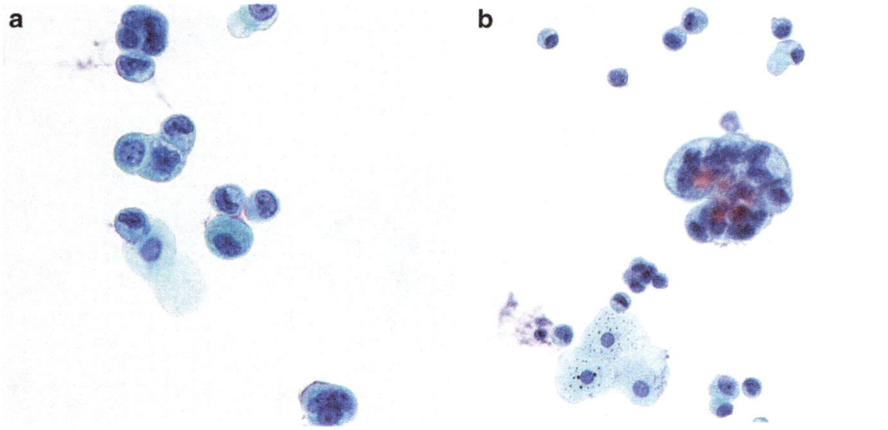

Fig. 4.6 Atypical urothelial cells (AUC). Atypical urothelial cells with high N/C ratios. (**a**) The image shows enlarged nuclei (compared to the neighboring benign urothelial cells) and mild nuclear contour irregularities. The chromatin is uniform and hypochromatic, precluding a diagnosis of SHGUC (*Bladder washing, TP, high mag.*). (**b**) Abnormal nuclear contours are present in a degenerated aggregate of urothelial cells. The cellular changes are worrisome, but the degree of degeneration precludes a definitive diagnosis. Degenerative cytoplasmic vacuolization is demonstrated (*Bladder washing, TP, intermediate mag.*)

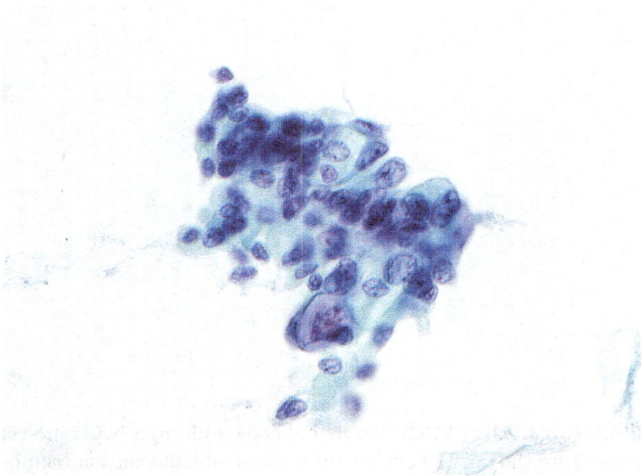

Fig. 4.7 Atypical urothelial cells (AUC). Urothelial cells with high N/C ratios display enlarged nuclei and conspicuous nuclear contour irregularity. The chromatin is clumped yet hypochromatic, precluding a diagnosis of SHGUC. (*Bladder Barbotage, ThinPrep, high mag.*)

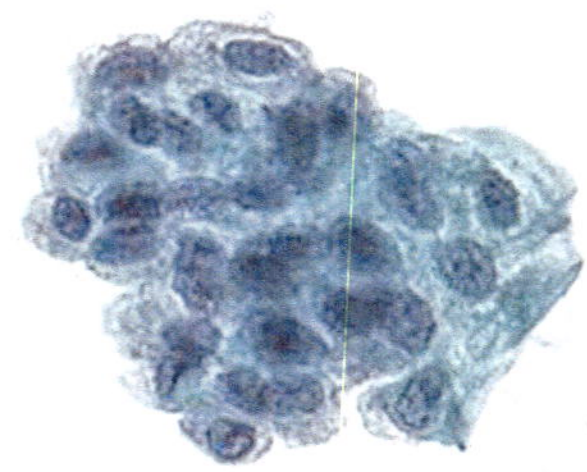

Fig. 4.8 Atypical urothelial cells (AUC). Urothelial cells with high N/C ratio, and nuclear hyperchromasia. Due to the degeneration, it is difficult to ascertain further chromatinic detail, therefore precluding a diagnosis of SHGUC. (*Voided urine, TP, high mag.*)

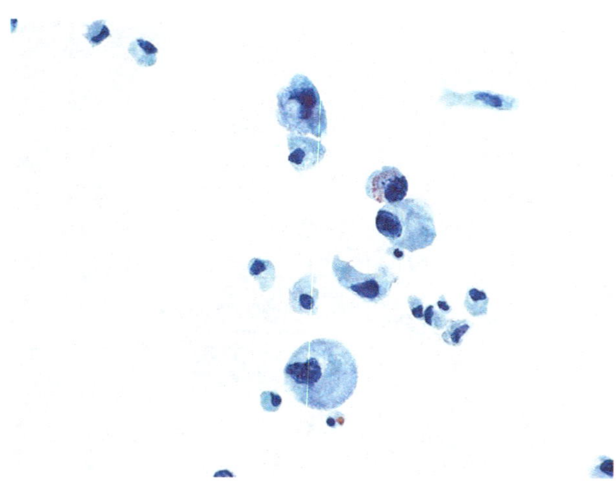

Fig. 4.9 Atypical urothelial cells (AUC). Urothelial cells with high N/C ratio (up to 50 %), and nuclear hyperchromasia are shown. The chromatin is coarse and the nuclear membranes are irregular. While the features are worrisome for high grade urothelial carcinoma, due to extensive degeneration and N/C ratio being less than 70 %, AUC diagnosis may be more appropriate. Follow up showed high grade urothelial carcinoma in the kidney; the urinary bladder had no pathology. (*Bladder washing, TP, high mag.*)

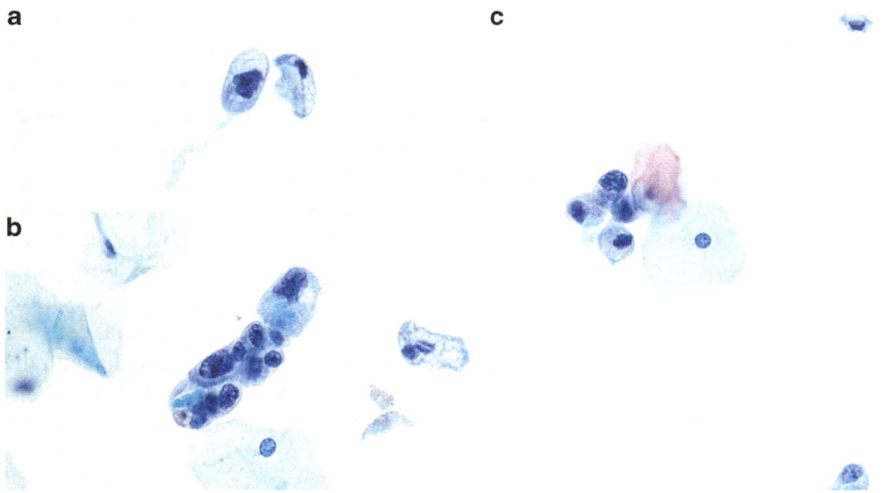

Fig. 4.10 Atypical urothelial cells (AUC). Urothelial cells with high N/C ratios, and nuclear hyperchromasia. (**a**) Atypical urothelial cell (AUC) (*upper left*). Urothelial cell displays irregular nuclear contours. (**b**) Group of urothelial cells with markedly irregular nuclear contours and variation in nuclear size (*lower left*). In comparison to the neighboring squamous cells there is mild nuclear hyperchromasia. There are degenerative cellular changes, such as partial loss of the cytoplasm and loss of crisp nuclear detail. (**c**) Small aggregate of atypical urothelial cells adjacent to squamous cells (*right*). The urothelial cell nuclei also show degeneration, but the one cell with the high N/C ratio is worrisome for carcinoma. The patient is a 36-year-old woman with recurrent urolithiasis, and no history of urothelial carcinoma. Her age and history are low-risk factors for bladder cancer. These three figures display the entire amount of atypical cells that are present in the specimen; therefore, these cytologic features warrant the diagnosis AUC (*Voided, TP, high mag.*)

minor criterion (the presence of two or more minor criteria, including hyperchromasia is diagnostic of SHGUC, unless there are marked degenerative changes):

- Major criterion (required)
  - Non-superficial and non-degenerated urothelial cells with an increased nuclear cytoplasmic (N/C) ratio (>0.5) (Explanatory Note 1)
- Minor criteria (one required):
  - Nuclear hyperchromasia (Explanatory Note 2)
  - Irregular nuclear membranes (chromatinic rim or nuclear contour) (Explanatory Note 3)
  - Irregular, coarse, clumped chromatin

Based on the presence of the one major criterion and one of the minor criteria noted above, a diagnosis of AUC may be rendered. Normal intermediate and basal urothelial cells, typically observed in instrumented urine specimens, should be identified and categorized as "normal" or NHGUC despite the fact that they have a high N/C ratio and may appear mildly hyperchromatic (Fig. 4.1). These cells frequently occur in groups, show uniform, round nuclei and inconspicuous nucleoli with finely dispersed, smooth chromatin (see Chap. 3).

When the above-mentioned criteria are not met, factors such as poor cellular preservation (cellular degeneration), autolysis, obscuring blood, inflammatory cells, crystals, or hypocellularity may prevent a definitive diagnosis; an inadequate or unsatisfactory designation is prudent. The diagnosis of AUC is appropriate when criteria of the cells are more abnormal than NHGUC. In cases where there is a suspicion for HGUC, but there is also extensive degeneration, AUC is a valid choice.

Both the quality and quantity of AUC in a urine specimen are important for the diagnosis. In a recent study reviewing the subclassification of AUC, cases with a negative outcome had an average of less than 9 AUC, compared to cases with a tissue-confirmed HGUC outcome in which >16 AUC were present [3]. At this time, there is no recommendation for counting the number of atypical urothelial cells for an AUC diagnosis. However, it is clear that as the number of atypical cells with the described features increases so does the possibility of malignancy and the likelihood of the case being diagnosed as SHGUC or HGUC rather than AUC.

Explanatory Notes

Explanatory Note 1: *High N/C ratio*. HGUC cells often show a high N/C ratio exceeding 0.7 (meaning 70 % of the area of the cell is occupied by the nucleus). For a diagnosis of AUC, the N/C ratio should be at least 0.5 (50 %). If this is the sole finding, the case should not be reported under the AUC category.

Explanatory Note 2: *Nuclear hyperchromasia*. Hyperchromasia refers to an increased density of the nuclear chromatin of urothelial cells as compared with that of normal superficial urothelial cells (preferably) or intermediate squamous cells. Hyperchromasia reflects increased light absorption, resulting from increased chromatin density and affinity for nuclear dyes, variably seen in neoplastic cells. The staining intensity and texture of the nuclear chromatin should not be so pronounced as that of cells in the SHGUC or HGUC categories.

Explanatory Note 3: *Irregular nuclear membrane*. Compared with the round shape and smooth contours of the nuclei of normal urothelial cells, AUC usually show an irregular nuclear shape and variably thickened chromatinic rim, while still retaining a generally round, not oval, shape.

Other features that may be present in AUC:

Eccentric nuclei, in cells without columnar features, are usually a sign of loss of nuclear polarity: Urothelial cells with eccentric nuclei and high N/C ratios may raise the suspicion of malignancy. The differential diagnosis of such cells with eccentric nuclei includes native type of glandular cells (cystitis glandularis) and reactive renal tubular cells, which lack hyperchromasia, nuclear membrane irregularity, and irregular clumped chromatin. Cases in which eccentric nuclei are the sole finding should not be reported as AUC.

Presence of urothelial cell clusters in voided urine specimens: The mere presence of benign clusters in voided urine specimens does not fulfill the criteria for AUC, unless the urothelial cells within the group also show two of the described cytologic criteria (one major and one minor; see above).

Large nuclear size: The nucleus of AUC cells is usually larger than that of intermediate or basal urothelial cells, intermediate squamous cells, or benign columnar cells. However, decreased or normal-appearing nuclear size can be associated with cellular shrinkage and may occasionally be seen in cells otherwise fulfilling the diagnostic criteria for AUC.

Rate and Risk of Malignancy

The reporting rate of atypia ranges from 2 to 31 % (Table 4.1). To date there hasn't been a uniform, standardized description of AUC. Once strict criteria are utilized, the rate of atypia should decrease. Despite the efforts to define this category as narrowly as possible and to provide specific morphologic criteria, an AUC diagnosis will have only fair reproducibility, just like its counterpart in reporting cytologic samples from the thyroid [4] and gynecologic tract [5]. However, in order to preserve the credibility of this diagnosis, the frequency of an AUC interpretation should be minimized similar to that of the "atypical" categories of other reporting systems such as The Bethesda System for Reporting Thyroid Cytology. As further studies are performed utilizing the criteria set forth in The Paris System and as more evidence-based data become available, recommendations for the frequency of AUC interpretation will evolve.

The risk of detecting a biopsy-proven HGUC following an AUC diagnosis ranges from 8.3 to 37.5 % (see Table 4.1). These rates are usually inversely proportional to the institutional rate of AUC diagnoses, and may depend on the interval between the cytological and histological diagnoses. Historically, the follow-up of patients with AUC diagnoses has shown a wide spectrum of conditions, from benign diseases (urolithiasis, cystitis, benign prostatic hypertrophy, renal disease, diabetes mellitus, irradiation, intravesical chemotherapy, BCG immunotherapy, recent TUR, indwelling catheter, post-instrumentation, inverted papilloma, hyperplasia, nephrogenic adenoma, etc.) to malignant diseases (HGUC or LGUC).

Table 4.1 Published reporting rates and the follow-up of atypical urothelial cells

Study	Year	Rate of AUC (%)	Follow-up HGUC (%)
Barasch et al. [6]	2013	5.7	14.3
Rosenthal et al. [7]	2013	31.0	18.0
Piaton et al. [8]	2014	<2	8.3
Muus et al. [9]	2012	8.1	21.0
Mokhtar et al. [10]	2010	2.1	37.5
Brimo et al. [11]	2009	26.0	37.0
Streeter et al. [12]	2008	N/A	30.9
Kapur et al. [13]	2008	6.9	33.0
Bhatia et al. [14]	2006	1.9	20.0
Deshpande et al. [15]	2005	N/A	13.0

AUC Atypical urothelial cells, *HGUC* high-grade urothelial carcinoma, *N/A* not applicable

Since the main aim of urine cytology is to detect HGUC, a diagnosis of "atypia" is inappropriate for known benign conditions such as reactive umbrella cells, viral changes due to polyomavirus or other viruses, granulomas, or changes due to urolithiasis as discussed in Chap. 3 [2]. With the current, stricter definition of AUC, the follow-up of patients with this diagnosis is expected to change. On one hand, the exclusion from this category of cell groups without cytologic atypia and of "atypia" associated with known causes is expected to result in a higher proportion of benign (NHGUC) not neoplastic conditions. On the other hand, since this reporting system also includes a well-defined "suspicious" category (SHGUC), some cases formerly interpreted as AUC will be interpreted as SHGUC, potentially resulting in a lower proportion of HGUC in the follow-up of AUC. (For further discussion see Chap. 5.)

References

1. Pambuccian SE. What is atypia? Use, misuse and overuse of the term atypia in diagnostic cytopathology. J Am Soc Cytopathol. 2015;4:44–52.
2. Wojcik EM. What should not be reported as atypia in urine cytology. J Am Soc Cytopathol. 2015;4:30–6.
3. McCroskey Z, Bahar B, Hu Z, Wojcik EM, Barkan GA. Subclassifying atypia in urine cytology: what are the helpful features? J Am Soc Cytopathol. 2015;4:183–9.
4. Cochand-Priollet B, Schmitt FC, Tötsch M, Vielh P, European Federation of Cytology Societies' Scientific Committee. The Bethesda terminology for reporting thyroid cytopathology: from theory to practice in Europe. Acta Cytol. 2011;55:507–11.
5. Sherman ME, Dasgupta A, Schiffman M, Nayar R, Solomon D. The Bethesda Interobserver Reproducibility Study (BIRST): a web-based assessment of the Bethesda 2001 System for classifying cervical cytology. Cancer. 2007;111:15–25.
6. Barasch S, Choi M, Stewart III J, Das K. Significance of atypical category in voided urine specimens prepared by liquid-based technology: experience of a single institution. J Am Soc Cytopathol. 2014;3:118–25.
7. Rosenthal DL, VandenBussche CJ, Burroughs FH, Sathiyamoorthy S, Guan H, Owens C. The Johns Hopkins Hospital template for urologic cytology samples: part I-creating the template. Cancer Cytopathol. 2013;121:15–20.
8. Piaton E, Decaussin-Petrucci M, Mege-Lechevallier F, Advenier AS, Devonec M, Ruffion A. Diagnostic terminology for urinary cytology reports including the new subcategories 'atypical urothelial cells of undetermined significance' (AUC-US) and 'cannot exclude high grade' (AUC-H). Cytopathology. 2014;25:27–38.
9. Muus Ubago J, Mehta V, Wojcik EM, Barkan GA. Evaluation of atypical urine cytology progression to malignancy. Cancer Cytopathol. 2013;121:387–91.
10. Mokhtar GA, Al-Dousari M, Al-Ghamedi D. Diagnostic significance of atypical category in the voided urine samples: a retrospective study in a tertiary care center. Urol Ann. 2010;2:100–6.
11. Brimo F, Vollmer RT, Case B, Aprikian A, Kassouf W, Auger M. Accuracy of urine cytology and the significance of an atypical category. Am J Clin Pathol. 2009;132:785–93.
12. Streeter EH, Turner GD, McCormick R, Roberts IS, Crew J. The significance of atypical urine cytology in the face of normal investigations—is extended investigation and follow-up required? Br J Med Surg Urol. 2008;1:131–5.
13. Kapur U, Venkataraman G, Wojcik EM. Diagnostic significance of 'atypia' in instrumented versus voided urine specimens. Cancer. 2008;114:270–4.
14. Bhatia A, Dey P, Kakkar N, Srinivasan R, Nijhawan R. Malignant atypical cell in urine cytology: a diagnostic dilemma. Cytojournal. 2006;3:28.
15. Deshpande V, McKee GT. Analysis of atypical urine cytology in a tertiary care center. Cancer. 2005;105:468–75.

Chapter 5
Suspicious for High-Grade Urothelial Carcinoma (Suspicious)

Fadi Brimo, Manon Auger, Tarik M. Elsheikh, Hui Guan, Mitsuru Kinjo, Eric Piaton, Dorothy L. Rosenthal, Tatsuro Shimokama, and Rosemary H. Tambouret

Background

The diagnosis of "suspicious for HGUC" (SHGUC) is meant to reflect the presence of urothelial cells with severe atypia that falls short for a diagnosis of high-grade urothelial carcinoma (HGUC), but beyond atypia that is associated with the "atypical urothelial cells" (AUC) category. Although this term has not been consistently used in the literature, terminologies such as "AUC cannot exclude HGUC or AUC-H"; "AUC, favor malignant" and "suspicious for malignancy" have been reported in the same context in order to convey similar degrees of concern and uncertainty to the treating physician [1–6]. Studies investigating the significance of this cytological diagnosis are rare, and while some used nonspecific descriptive criteria, others in which well-defined criteria were reported did not necessarily use the term "SHGUC" by applying the same qualitative and/or quantitative morphological features. This has resulted in interinstitutional variations in the rate of this diagnosis as well as its association with a subsequent histological diagnosis of HGUC that has precluded generating unifying clinical guidelines in following or treating patients with a "SHGUC" cytological result.

Definition

This diagnosis is restrictively used in cases with abnormal urothelial cells that quantitatively fall short of a definitive diagnosis of HGUC.

D.L. Rosenthal et al. (eds.), *The Paris System for Reporting Urinary Cytology*,
DOI 10.1007/978-3-319-22864-8_5

Criteria

A diagnosis of "SHGUC" (Figs. 5.1, 5.2, 5.3, 5.4, 5.5, 5.6, 5.7, 5.8, and 5.9) is defined as non-superficial and non-degenerated urothelial cells showing:

- Increased nuclear to cytoplasmic (N/C) ratio, at least 0.5–0.7 "Required diagnostic criterion"
- Moderate to severe hyperchromasia "Required diagnostic criterion"

In addition, at least one of the two following features needs to be present:

- Irregular clumpy chromatin
- Marked irregular nuclear membranes

Using all the features listed above, the decision to assign the case into the "SHGUC" or the "positive for HGUC" categories is based on the number of the abnormal cells fulfilling the above criteria. Depending on individual cases assigned to the "suspicious" category, the number of abnormal cells can range from as low as one to as high as ten cells. Due to the lack of definitive data derived from studies specifically addressing this quantitative issue, a strict cut-off number of abnormal cells above which one can confidently assign a "positive for HGUC" diagnosis cannot be definitely implemented at the current time. Instead, a cut-off range of 5–10 cells is recommended based on the degree of abnormal nuclear changes observed, and the level of pathologist's comfort. Accordingly, a "positive for HGUC" diagnosis should very rarely, if ever, be assigned in the presence of less than five abnormal

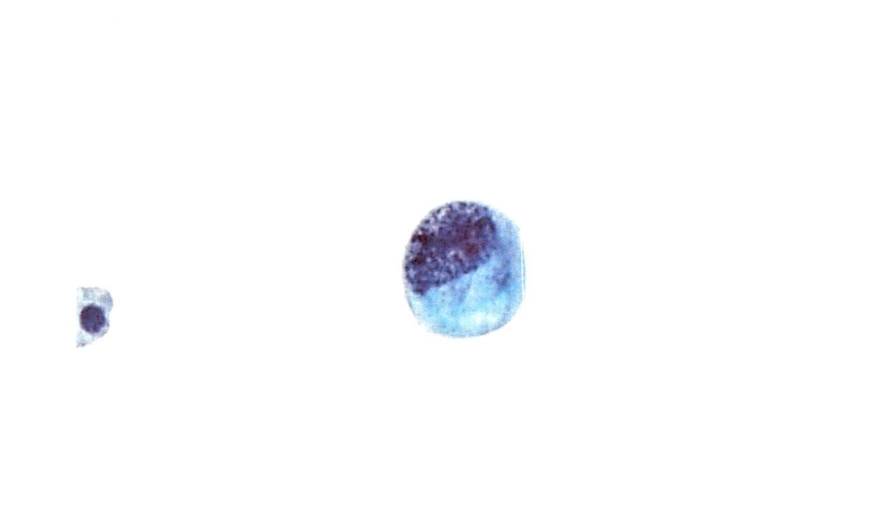

Fig. 5.1 Suspicious for high-grade urothelial carcinoma (SHGUC). One single abnormal well-preserved intermediate urothelial cell displays an eccentric nucleus with increased N/C ratio, hyperchromasia, irregular clumpy chromatin, and mildly irregular nuclear membrane (*Voided urine, TP, high mag.*)

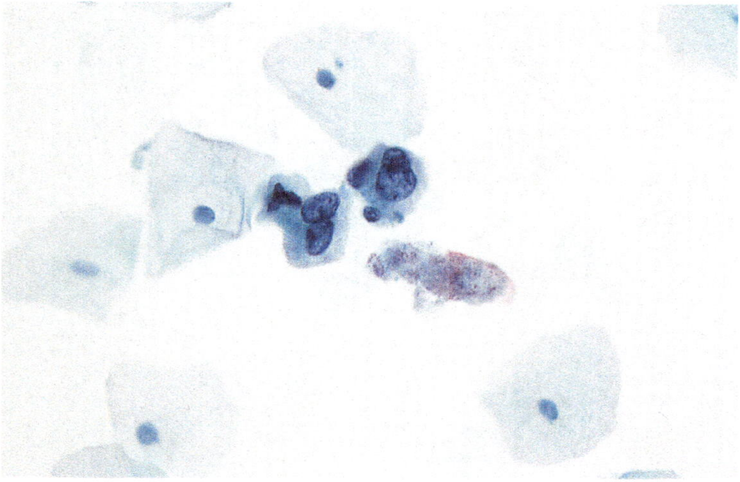

Fig. 5.2 Suspicious for high-grade urothelial carcinoma (SHGUC). Rare but abnormal well-preserved intermediate urothelial cells showing increased N/C ratios, hyperchromasia, and irregular nuclear membranes (*Catheterized urine, CS, high mag.*)

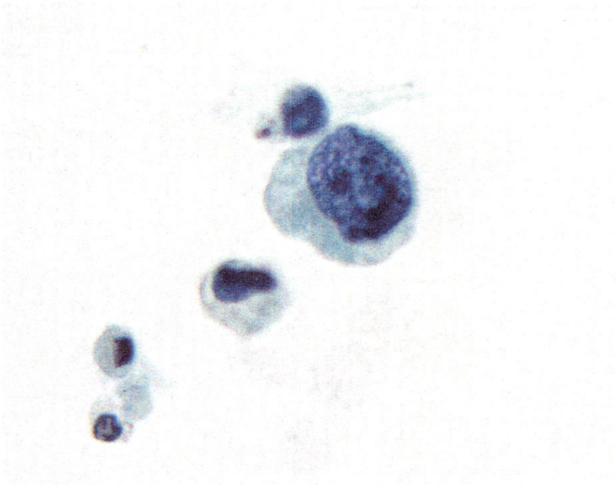

Fig. 5.3 Suspicious for high-grade urothelial carcinoma (SHGUC). A few abnormal intermediate urothelial cells, one of which is well preserved (center) and features an increased N/C ratio, hyperchromasia, irregular clumpy chromatin, and severely irregular nuclear membrane. If more than five similar cells were found, the diagnosis of HGUC would be appropriate (*Catheterized urine, CS, high mag.*)

well-preserved cells. In comparison, in the presence of 5–10 abnormal cells, the decision to assign a "positive for HGUC" diagnosis should take into account the severity of atypia of all the abnormal cells, the clinical context as well as the specimen

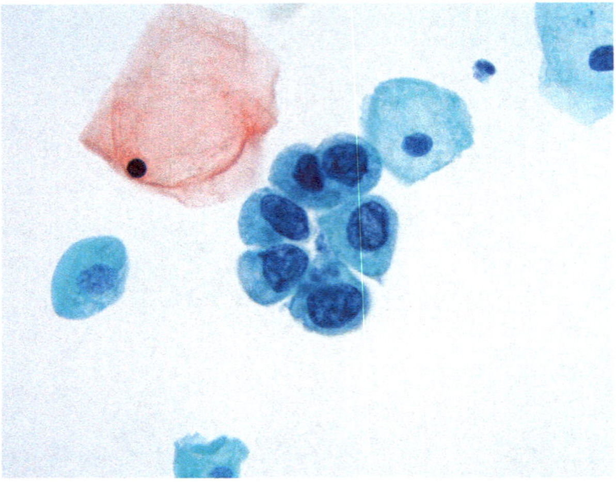

Fig. 5.4 Suspicious for high-grade urothelial carcinoma (SHGUC). A cell cluster composed of six abnormal well-preserved intermediate urothelial cells showing increased N/C ratios, hyperchromasia, clumpy chromatin, and irregular nuclear membranes. Note that not all the cells have an N/C ratio that exceeds 0.7 but in the presence of similar nuclear characteristics, they should be considered part of the same lesion. A "positive for HGUC" diagnosis may be acceptable in this case, especially in the presence of a previous history of HGUC (*Catheterized urine, CS, high mag.*)

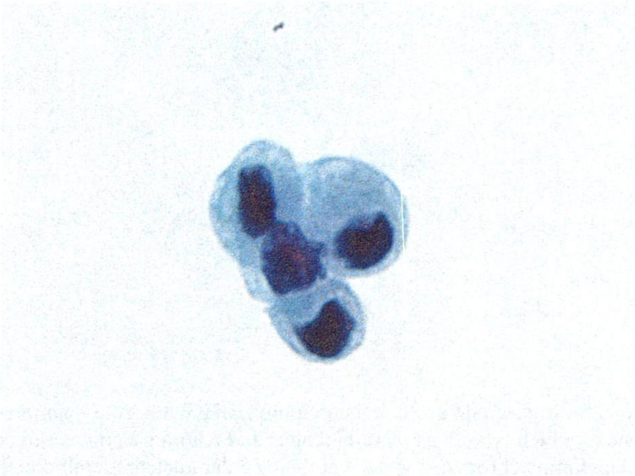

Fig. 5.5 Suspicious for high-grade urothelial carcinoma (SHGUC). A cell cluster composed of four abnormal well-preserved intermediate urothelial cells having increased N/C ratios, hyperchromasia, and irregular nuclear membranes in the absence of clear chromatin details. Note that the N/C ratios vary significantly within the group with only two cells having an N/C ratio exceeding 0.7 (*Voided urine, TP, high mag.*)

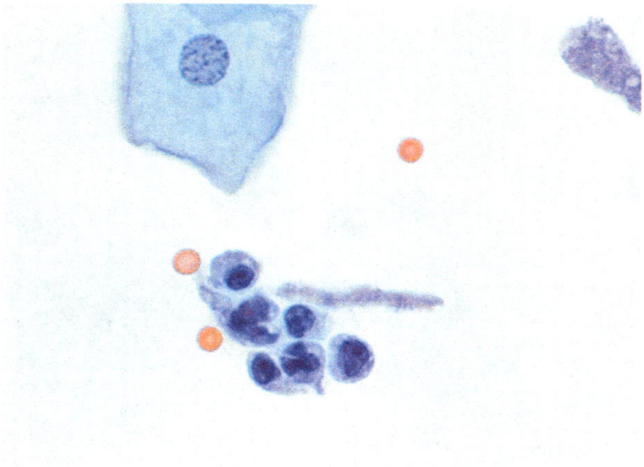

Fig. 5.6 Suspicious for high-grade urothelial carcinoma (SHGUC). A few abnormal well-preserved intermediate urothelial cells display increased N/C ratios, hyperchromasia, prominent nucleoli, and irregular nuclear membranes in the absence of evaluable chromatin details (*Catheterized urine, CS, high mag.*)

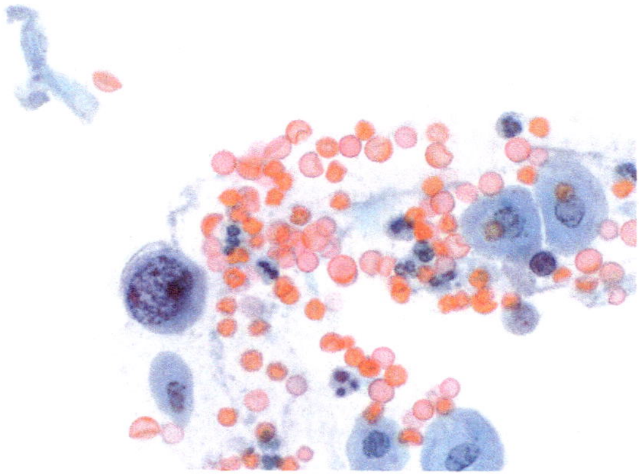

Fig. 5.7 Suspicious for high-grade urothelial carcinoma (SHGUC). One single abnormal well-preserved intermediate urothelial cell showing increased N/C ratio, hyperchromasia, irregular clumpy chromatin, and smooth regular nuclear membranes. Note the severe hyperchromasia in comparison to the normal intermediate urothelial cells (*right*) (*Catheterized urine, CS, high mag.*)

type. As an example, in the presence of a previous history of HGUC and/or in voided specimens which are by nature less cellular than instrumented specimens and in which cellular degeneration is frequent, as low as five well-preserved and severely abnormal cells with the features listed above may be sufficient to render a definitive "positive for HGUC" diagnosis. On the other hand, it is recommended to have at least ten abnormal cells before labelling a case as "positive for HGUC" in

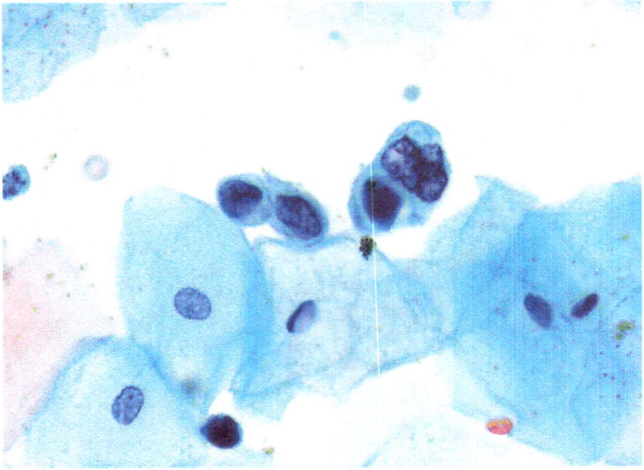

Fig. 5.8 Suspicious for high-grade urothelial carcinoma (SHGUC). Rare but abnormal well-preserved intermediate urothelial cells having increased N/C ratios, hyperchromasia, clumpy chromatin, and irregular nuclear membranes. Note that although the nuclear size is not significantly larger than normal intermediate cell nuclei, the cells contain cytological nuclear abnormalities that warrant a "suspicious for high-grade urothelial carcinoma" diagnosis (*Voided urine, SP, high mag.*)

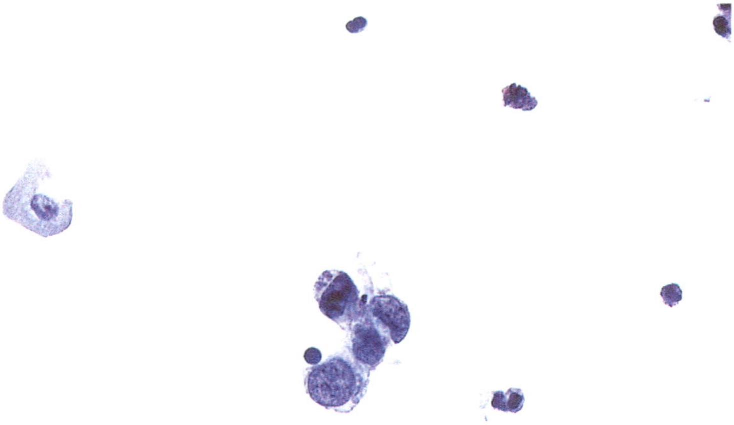

Fig. 5.9 Suspicious for high-grade urothelial carcinoma (SHGUC). Rare but abnormal well-preserved intermediate urothelial cells showing increased N/C ratios, hyperchromasia, irregular nuclear membranes but overall fine evenly distributed chromatin (*Voided urine, TP, medium mag.*)

instrumented specimens derived from the upper urothelial tract (see Chap. 6, for further discussion).

- The cells are usually seen as single cells although clusters of atypical cells may also be present. The above diagnostic criteria are most reliably assessed in the single cells.

- Nuclear size is usually at least twice the size of the normal intermediate or deep cell's nucleus although this feature is not mandatory.
- Features that may be seen but do not necessarily need to be present are:
  - Eccentric nuclear location (see Fig. 5.1).
  - Necrotic background.
  - Pleomorphism.
  - Mitoses.
  - Apoptotic bodies.

Explanatory Notes

Explanatory Note 1: Increased N/C ratio generally refers to an enlarged nucleus that occupies at least half of the surface of the cell provided the cell is not degenerated and the cytoplasm is complete. In the vast majority of cases falling into the "suspicious" category, the N/C ratio of the abnormal cell exceeds 0.7 and it is recommended to have at least one of the abnormal cells in the specimen showing such marked N/C ratio increase. This being said, since the evaluation of the N/C ratio by visual inspection can be subjective and since an N/C ratio exceeding 0.7 is not necessarily present in all the cells of high-grade urothelial lesions even in histological specimens, the cut-off of 0.7 should not be used with strictness and the final decision to assign a "suspicious" diagnosis should take into account the specimen's type, clinical history, the degree of nuclear atypia of the abnormal cells, and the N/C ratio of the other abnormal cells. As an example, a "suspicious" diagnosis may sometimes still be acceptable even if the N/C ratio of the abnormal cells is between 0.5 and 0.7 provided the cells show the other described associated abnormal cytological features (see Figs. 5.1 and 5.5). The latter approach is especially acceptable in voided specimens or in patients known to have a previous history of HGUC. In comparison, as instrumentation is usually associated with an increased N/C ratio even in the benign urothelial cells, it is recommended to use the cut-off of 0.7 in non-voided specimens.

Explanatory Note 2: Hyperchromasia refers to an increased density of the nuclear chromatin of abnormal urothelial cells as compared with that of the normal umbrella or intermediate urothelial cells. It is required that the degree of hyperchromasia be moderate to severe; a mild difference in the chromatin density between the abnormal urothelial cell assessed and the normal accompanying cells does not warrant a "suspicious" diagnosis (Fig. 5.10).

Explanatory Note 3: In the absence of clear and evaluable chromatin details, the irregular clumpy chromatin pattern is not required in the presence of the other three features (high N/C ratio, irregular nuclear membranes, hyperchromasia) (see Fig. 5.6). Similarly, the presence of nuclear membrane irregularity is not required in the presence of the other three features (increased N/C ratio, hyperchromasia, irregular clumpy chromatin) (see Fig. 5.7).

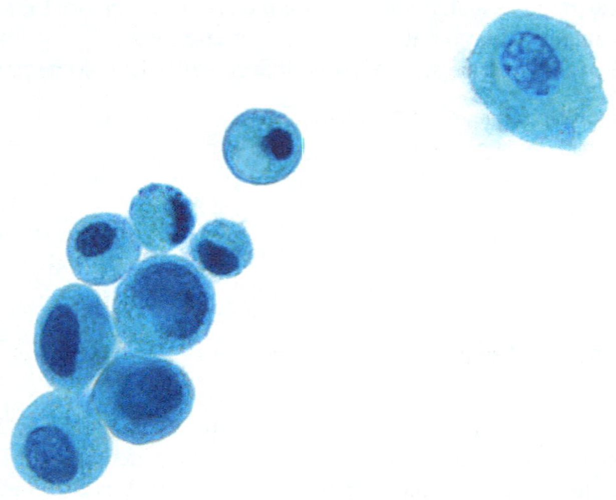

Fig. 5.10 Atypical urothelial cells (AUC). Cell clusters of well-preserved intermediate urothelial cells some of which show an increased N/C ratio and hyperchromasia. The degree of hyperchromasia is mild in comparison to the normal intermediate cell nucleus (*upper right*). In addition, the cells do not show clumpy chromatin pattern or irregular nuclear membranes which preclude the assignment of a SHGUC diagnosis (*Voided urine, TP, high mag.*)

Explanatory Note 4: Intermediate urothelial cells with increased N/C ratio and mild hyperchromasia and/or in the absence of evaluable chromatin details and irregular nuclear membranes should not be labelled as "suspicious" but as "AUC" instead. Similarly, cells with increased N/C ratio and irregular nuclear membranes in the absence of severe hyperchromasia should be labelled as "AUC" rather than "suspicious" (Figs. 5.11 and 5.12).

Explanatory Note 5: While the category of "AUC" includes a subset of cases showing cellular degeneration, a "SHGUC" diagnosis should not be rendered on degenerated cells. Cellular degeneration is often present in voided specimens and can take the form of incomplete cytoplasm, poorly preserved chromatin details, or discontinuous nuclear membranes. The resulting altered cellular morphology can be problematic from the diagnostic standpoint for the following reasons:

- Nuclei may look "blown-up" resulting in a falsely increased N/C ratio (Figs. 5.13 and 5.14).
- Cytoplasm may be incomplete which makes it difficult to assess the N/C ratio (see Fig. 5.14b).
- Nuclear membranes may seem irregular from dehydration.
- Nucleus may look hyperchromatic as a feature of degeneration, and not as a result of an abnormal chromatin (see Figs. 5.13 and 5.14).

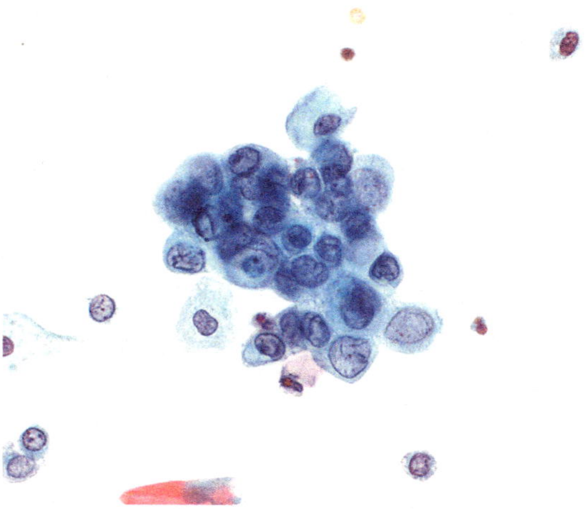

Fig. 5.11 Atypical urothelial cells (AUC). Abnormal intermediate urothelial cells showing increased N/C ratio and irregular nuclear membranes in the absence of nuclear hyperchromasia preclude a diagnosis of SHGUC. The follow-up diagnosis was LGUC (*Voided urine, TP, high mag.*)

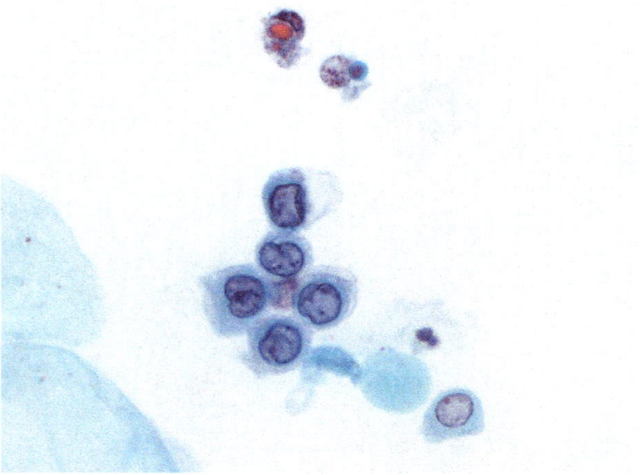

Fig. 5.12 Atypical urothelial cells (AUC). Abnormal intermediate urothelial cells displaying increased N/C ratio and irregular nuclear membranes in the absence of nuclear hyperchromasia preclude a diagnosis of SHGUC (*Voided urine, TP, high mag.*)

Explanatory Note 6: The presence of prominent nucleoli is not a definitive feature of malignancy as it can be seen in reactive urothelial cells. Reactive urothelial cells may have an increased N/C ratio bordering on and sometimes exceeding 0.5 but have regular nuclear membranes and fine chromatin provided they are well preserved (Fig. 5.15).

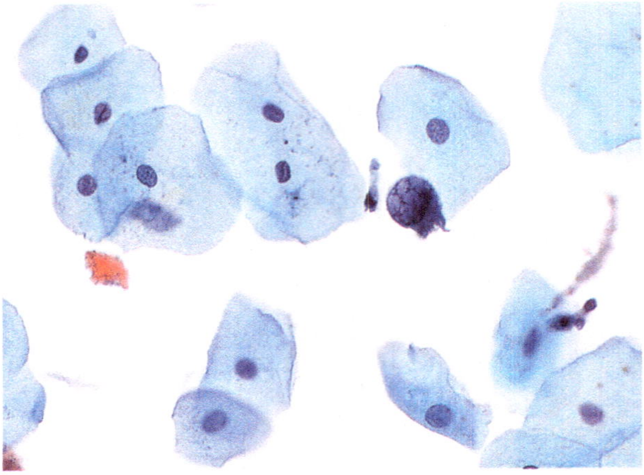

Fig. 5.13 Atypical urothelial cells (AUC). One single and degenerated urothelial cell showing enlarged nucleus, increased N/C ratio, mild hyperchromasia, and irregularly distributed clumpy chromatin. Note the presence of incomplete cytoplasm and poorly preserved chromatin details. A "suspicious for high-grade urothelial carcinoma" diagnosis should not be rendered on degenerated cells. In this case, polyomavirus infection may also be considered and a negative diagnosis may be appropriate (*Voided urine, TP, high mag.*)

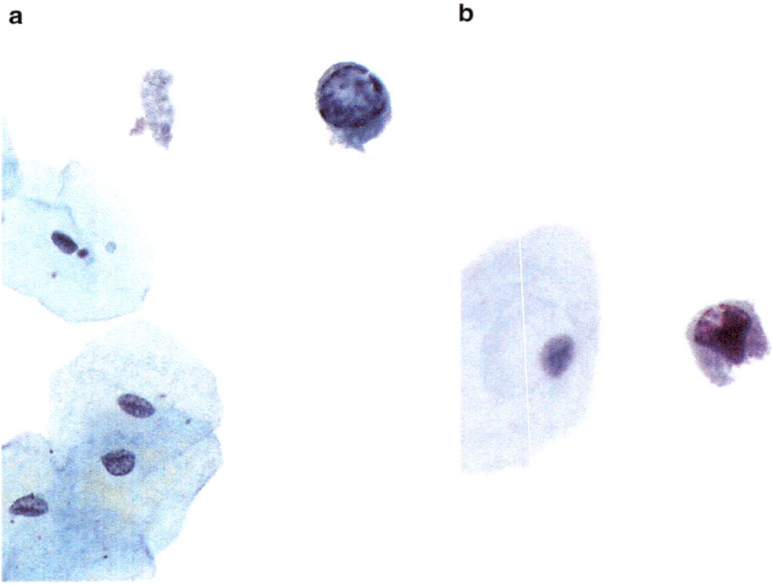

Fig. 5.14 (**a**) Atypical urothelial cells (AUC). One single and degenerated urothelial cell showing increased N/C ratio, hyperchromasia, and irregularly distributed clumpy chromatin. Note the presence of incomplete cytoplasm and discontinuous nuclear membranes. In the presence of cellular degeneration a SHGUC diagnosis should not be rendered (*Voided urine, TP, high mag.*) (**b**) Atypical urothelial cells (AUC). One single and degenerated urothelial cell showing increased N/C ratio, hyperchromasia, and irregularly distributed clumpy chromatin. Note the presence of incomplete cytoplasm and discontinuous nuclear membranes. In the presence of cellular degeneration a "suspicious for high-grade urothelial carcinoma" diagnosis should not be rendered (*Voided urine, TP, high mag.*)

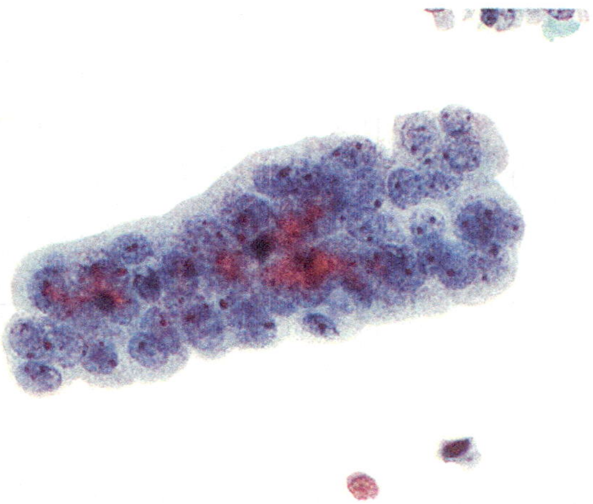

Fig. 5.15 Negative for malignancy. Cells clusters of well-preserved intermediate urothelial cells have increased N/C ratios. However, hyperchromasia is absent and the nuclei show fine regularly distributed chromatin with small visible nucleoli. Nuclear membranes are smooth and regular (*Voided urine, TP, high mag.*)

Rate and Risk of Malignancy

This information is limited by the scarcity of related studies in which well-defined morphological criteria were used that would enable accurate and meaningful data comparison [2, 5–7] (Table 5.1). In the four largest studies conducted to date, the reported rates of a "SHGUC" diagnosis or its equivalent (AUC-H) range from 2 to 6 % (mean of 3.2 %). The risk of detecting a subsequent biopsy-proven high-grade urothelial lesion ranges from 37.8 to 95 % depending on the time frame between the cytological and the histological diagnoses. As an example, restricting the cytological–histological correlation to a period of 6 months or less shows predictive values ranging from 37.8 to 79 %. In comparison, correlating a "SHGUC" diagnosis with any subsequent histological result independent of the intervening period of time increases the yield of the "suspicious" cytological category to 80–95 %. In one of those studies, the performance of the "SHGUC" category was compared to that of "positive for HGUC" in terms of detecting high-grade lesions. In that study, a "positive" diagnosis showed closer associations with subsequent HGUC (predictive value of 86 % below 6 months and 90 % beyond 6 months interval) in comparison to a "suspicious" diagnosis (predictive value of 79 % below 6 months and 80 % beyond 6 months interval) (see Table 5.1).

Table 5.1 Comparison of the four largest studies evaluating the value of a "suspicious for HGUC" cytological diagnosis

Study	Number of patients	Rate (%)	Association with HGUC within 6 months	Association with HGUC beyond 6 months
Sternberg et al. [5]	111	3.2	N/A	61.3 % (up to 37 months f/u)
Ton Nu et al. [7]	447	2.5	79 %	80 % (up to 15 months f/u)
Piaton et al. [2]	185	2	37.8 %	88 % (up to 56 months f/u)
VandenBussche et al. [6]	62	6	N/A	95 % (up to 36 months f/u)

f/u follow-up, *HGUC* high-grade urothelial carcinoma, *N/A* not applicable

References

1. Brimo F, Vollmer RT, Case B, Aprikian A, Kassouf W, Auger M. Accuracy of urine cytology and the significance of an atypical category. Am J Clin Pathol. 2009;132:785–93.
2. Piaton E, Decaussin-Petrucci M, Mege-Lechevallier F, Advenier AS, Devonec M, Ruffion A. Diagnostic terminology for urinary cytology reports including the new subcategories 'atypical urothelial cells of undetermined significance' (AUC-US) and 'cannot exclude high grade' (AUC-H). Cytopathology. 2014;25:27–38.
3. Raitanen MP, Aine RA, Kaasinen ES, Liukkonen TJ, Kylmälä TM, Huhtala H, Tammela TL, Finnbladder Group. Suspicious urine cytology (class III) in patients with bladder cancer: should it be considered as negative or positive? Scand J Urol Nephrol. 2002;36:213–7.
4. Rosenthal DL, VandenBussche CJ, Burroughs FH, Sathiyamoorthy S, Guan H, Owens C. The Johns Hopkins Hospital template for urologic cytology samples: part I—creating the template. Cancer Cytopathol. 2013;121:5–20.
5. Sternberg I, Rona R, Olsfanger S, Lew S, Leibovitch I. The clinical significance of class III (suspicious) urine cytology. Cytopathology. 2011;22:329–33.
6. VandenBussche CJ, Sathiyamoorthy S, Owens CL, Burroughs FH, Rosenthal DL, Guan H. The Johns Hopkins Hospital template for urologic cytology samples: parts II and III: improving the predictability of indeterminate results in urinary cytologic samples: an outcomes and cytomorphologic study. Cancer Cytopathol. 2013;121:21–8.
7. Ton Nu TN, Kassouf W, Ahmadi-Kaliji B, Charbonneau M, Auger M, Brimo F. The value of the "suspicious for urothelial carcinoma" cytology category: a correlative study of 4 years including 337 patients. Cancer Cytopathol. 2014;122:796–803.

Chapter 6
High-Grade Urothelial Carcinoma (HGUC)

Momin T. Siddiqui, Guido Fadda, Jee-Young Han, Christopher L. Owens, Z. Laura Tabatabai, and Toyonori Tsuzuki

Background

Historical Review of Reporting System of Urine Cytology

Urine cytology is an important test for screening and diagnosis of newly developed urothelial carcinoma (UC) and for surveillance of UC recurrence and new neoplasms. Urine cytology has been used for a long time because of its merits such as easy availability and noninvasive testing, high sensitivity, and specificity for high-grade urothelial carcinoma (HGUC), and great effectiveness to evaluate the entire urothelial tract. With urine cytology, the high-grade malignant cells can be identified even in occult carcinoma that is not visible cystoscopically [1, 2]. Therefore, despite the low sensitivity for low-grade urothelial neoplasm (LGUN) and the development of several newer techniques such as fluorescence in situ hybridization (FISH) for screening and diagnosis of UC, urine cytology still remains the gold standard for bladder cancer screening, especially for HGUC.

The reporting system for urine cytology has evolved over a period of time according to the changes in the histopathologic classification of UC [3]. Initially, Dr. Papanicolaou suggested a reporting system of urine cytology that included five classes [4]. Although this reporting system had a great role in diagnosing high-grade UC, the definitions or criteria for each category were somewhat unclear [4]. On the basis of the histopathologic classification of bladder cancer by the 1973 World Health Organization (WHO) classification, Koss et al. reported a new classification scheme for urine cytology [5]. In this classification, HGUC was characterized by the presence of hyperchromasia and nuclear membrane abnormalities in the malignant cells. After changes in the histopathologic classification of UC by the WHO/International Society of Urological Pathology in 1998, the Papanicolaou Society of Cytopathology (PSC) Task Force also reported a diagnostic classification system for urine cytology similar

D.L. Rosenthal et al. (eds.), *The Paris System for Reporting Urinary Cytology*,
DOI 10.1007/978-3-319-22864-8_6

to the 2001 Bethesda System for reporting uterine cervical cytology [6, 7]. The PSC scheme identified three different and simplified categories: negative, positive, and an equivocal category, called atypical urothelial cells. For this category the authors proposed further studies to better establish criteria for subclassifying atypical specimens. The authors also addressed the incorporation of ancillary studies, such as FISH, into urine cytology reporting, reflecting the emergence of adjunctive studies in urine cytology that continues today. The PSC also suggested that a comment be included in the cytologic report to further classify the atypia as reactive or neoplastic. However, the criteria to separate reactive atypia from neoplastic atypia were not clearly defined.

The Meaning of Positive Urine Cytology

Urine cytology is more sensitive in detecting HGUC than LGUN. The sensitivity of urine cytology ranges from 10 to 43.6 % for low grade to 50–85 % for HGUC; and specificity ranges from 26.3 to 88 %, depending on the type of urine sample collection and type of clinical presentation [8, 9]. Positive urine cytology is clinically meaningful. In tumor recurrence of upper urinary tract UC, it has been found that HGUC recurred significantly earlier in the positive urine cytology group than in the negative urine cytology group [10]. Multivariate analysis also shows that gender, positive urine cytology, and tumor multifocality are independent risk factors for subsequent recurrence [10]. This suggests that positive urine cytology is significantly associated with the incidence of tumor recurrence and is independent of other clinicopathologic variables. Hence, positive urine cytology in primary upper urinary tract UC is valuable to predict prognosis, and preoperative positive urine cytology may be associated with higher prevalence of tumor recurrence [10]. Kobayashi et al. [11] have reported a relationship between positive urine cytology and tumor recurrence in the upper urinary tract UC. Positive urine cytology can be useful to predict tumor progression. Zieger et al. have reported that positive urine cytology is associated with tumor progression in patients with stage Ta UC [12]. Another study has reported that positive urine cytology shows significantly higher incidences of progression and cancer-specific mortality than negative urine cytology [13]. Koga et al. [14] described the progression rates of positive urine cytology group and negative urine cytology group, with 5-year cumulative incidences of 20 % and 2 %, respectively.

The Importance of Tumor Grade as a Prognostic Factor

Tumor grade is a strong prognostic factor. Tumor grade has a higher predictive value of tumor progression and mortality than tumor stage. The prognosis of urothelial tumors is influenced by grade than by stage if the tumors are the same grade. HGUC generally has a worse prognosis than LGUN, regardless of stage [15, 16]. Stage progression and mortality of UC are noted in as many as 65 % of patients with HGUC. The recurrence and tumor progression rates were 37 % and 40 %, respectively in patients ($n=85$) with Ta HGUC [16]. This suggests that tumor grade is highly correlated to recurrence, progression, and cancer-specific mortality.

The Cytologic Characteristics of HGUC

The cytomorphologic characteristics of HGUC have historically been described as follows: High nuclear to cytoplasmic (N/C) ratio, nuclear pleomorphism, nuclear margin irregularity, and hyperchromasia [4, 5, 17]. Chromatin abnormalities such as coarse clumping or homogenous chromatin pattern are also present. Comet, India-ink (single cells with deep black structureless nuclei) and apoptotic cells can also be noted. In addition, nuclear overlapping, and apoptosis are frequently observed in HGUC [17, 18]. In addition to these features, prominent nucleoli, isolated malignant cells and extensive necrosis are also characteristic features of HGUC in urine cytology specimens, with necrosis being an indicator for invasive disease [19].

Definition

Histologic Definition of HGUC

In the 2004 WHO classification, HGUC has papillary structures lined by tumor cells that are disorderly arranged and are cytologically malignant [20]. All tumors identical to grade 3 in the 1973 WHO classification, and some tumors of grade 2 in that classification belong to HGUC in the 2004 WHO classification [20]. The papillary fronds are frequently fused to each other. These tissue structures with abnormal cell characteristics and disorganized architecture are easily found at low scanning power. Pleomorphic nuclei with prominent nucleoli, if present, show loss of polarity and frequent mitoses. Carcinoma in situ (CIS) is frequently observed in the surrounding mucosa.

Histologic Definition of Carcinoma In Situ

CIS is grossly a flat lesion and composed of high-grade carcinoma cells which are cytologically malignant [20]. The morphologic criteria of CIS require the presence of severe cytologic pleomorphism. Full-thickness maturation arrest is not absolutely needed. The tumor cells are disorganized with loss of polarity and cohesiveness. The malignant cells are generally large and pleomorphic. Scant to abundant cytoplasm is present. The nucleus shows coarse or clumped chromatin. Prominent nucleoli are occasionally seen. Mitotic figures are frequently present.

Cytologic Definition of HGUC

Urine cytology cannot distinguish invasive HGUC from noninvasive HGUC or CIS. However, the background in CIS is reported to be clean without blood, abundant inflammation, and cell debris [21, 22]. The malignant cells usually display an N/C ratio that is 0.7 or greater, i.e., nucleus occupying more than 70 % of the cytoplasm, and demonstrate nuclear hyperchromasia, irregular nuclear membranes, and coarse chromatin (Figs. 6.1, 6.2, 6.3, 6.4, 6.5, 6.6, 6.7, and 6.8) [21, 22]. According to The Paris System consensus, a cellular cytologic urine specimen with a minimum of five to ten viable malignant cells will qualify as HGUC. The type of specimen and comfort level of the pathologist may contribute to the minimal number of abnormal cells required for a more definitive diagnosis of malignancy. For example, upper urinary tract instrumented specimens will require at least ten abnormal cells,

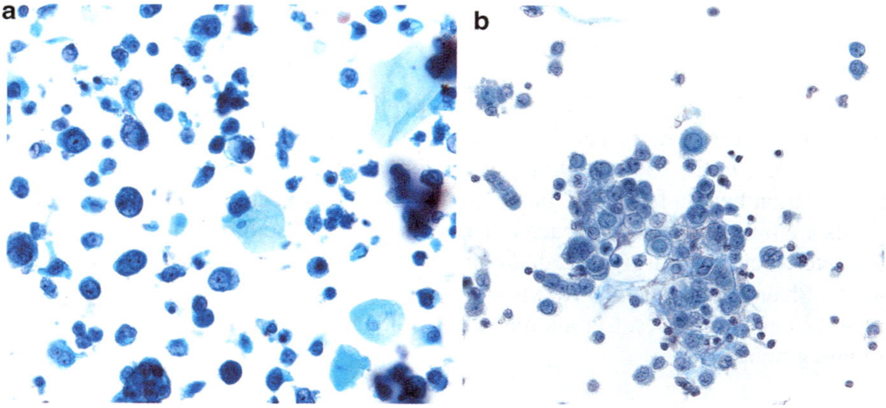

Fig. 6.1 High-grade urothelial carcinoma. (**a**) High-grade urothelial carcinoma (HGUC). The sample is hypercellular showing numerous tumor cells that demonstrate pleomorphism and necrosis in the background (*Voided urine, SP, low mag.*). (**b**) High-grade urothelial carcinoma (HGUC). The sample was full of these abnormal cells with high N/C ratios and prominent nuclear profiles. The total sample was stained somewhat lightly, so observers are cautioned to use normal cells in the background as stain intensity controls. Also note the presence of lymphocytes in the sample that can be used as controls for nuclear size (*Washing, TP, medium mag.*)

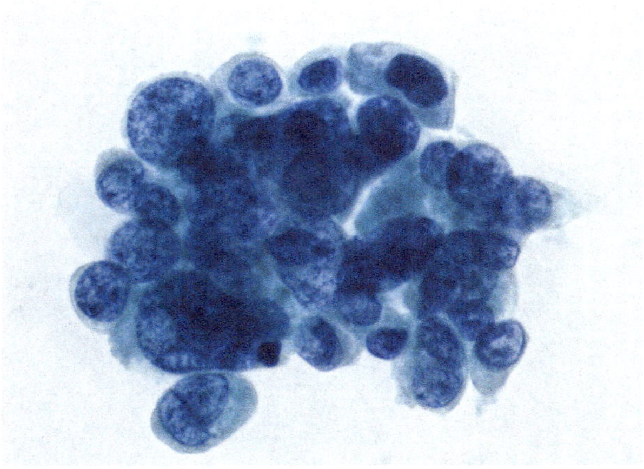

Fig. 6.2 High-grade urothelial carcinoma (HGUC) present as a cohesive group of malignant cells. The N/C ratio of 0.7 is noted in the majority of the tumor cells (*Bladder washing, TP, high mag.*)

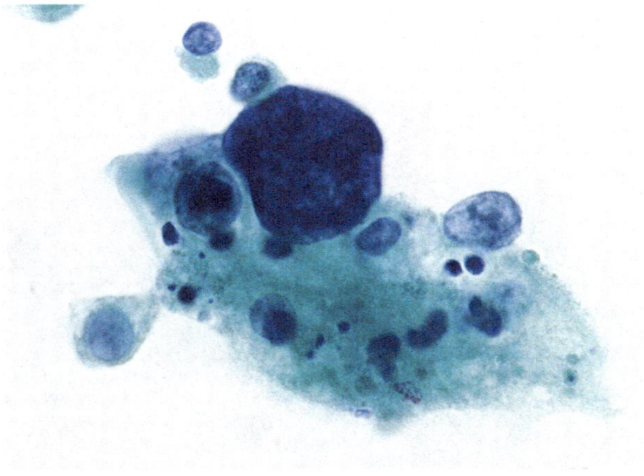

Fig. 6.3 Nuclear hyperchromasia is present in this cell from a patient with high-grade urothelial carcinoma (HGUC). Note the tumor necrosis clinging to the cells (*Bladder washing, TP, high mag.*)

whereas voided urine specimens may require a lesser number of cells to establish a definitive diagnosis of HGUC.

Definition of HGUC with Squamous Differentiation

This is defined by the presence of keratinization and/or intercellular bridges as classic morphological features. Squamous cells are intermixed with malignant cells exhibiting classic features of HGUC. The squamous cells display hyperchromatic

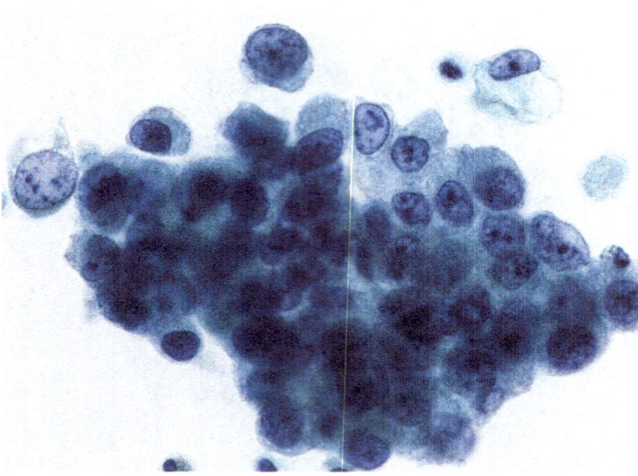

Fig. 6.4 High-grade urothelial carcinoma (HGUC) exhibits nuclear membrane irregularity with focal thickness of nuclear membranes. Nuclear shapes and sizes vary (*Bladder washing, TP, high mag.*)

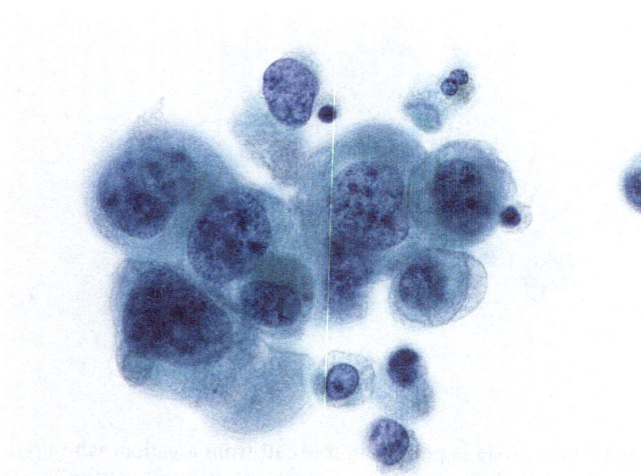

Fig. 6.5 High-grade urothelial carcinoma (HGUC) demonstrates coarse and clumped nuclear chromatin (*Voided Urine, TP, high mag.*)

and spindle-shaped nuclei with clumped chromatin. The cytoplasm is dense, keratinized, and orangeophilic. Keratin flakes and necrosis are frequently observed in the background (Figs. 6.9 and 6.10) [21–23]. Diagnosis of squamous carcinoma of the urinary tract can only be determined by extensive examination of biopsy or cystectomy tissue.

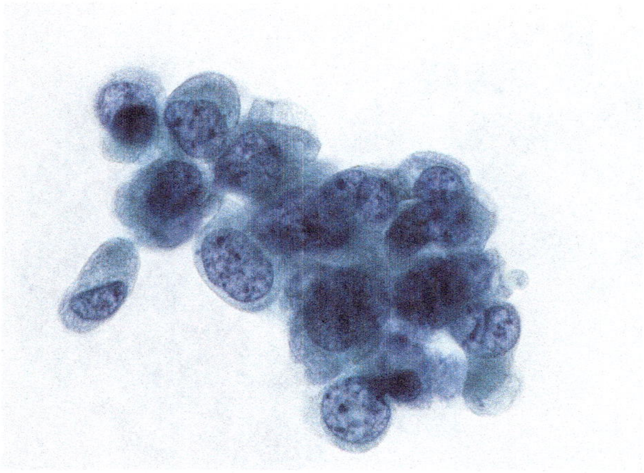

Fig. 6.6 High-grade urothelial carcinoma (HGUC) displays coarse chromatin and nuclear membrane irregularity (*Bladder washing, TP, high mag.*)

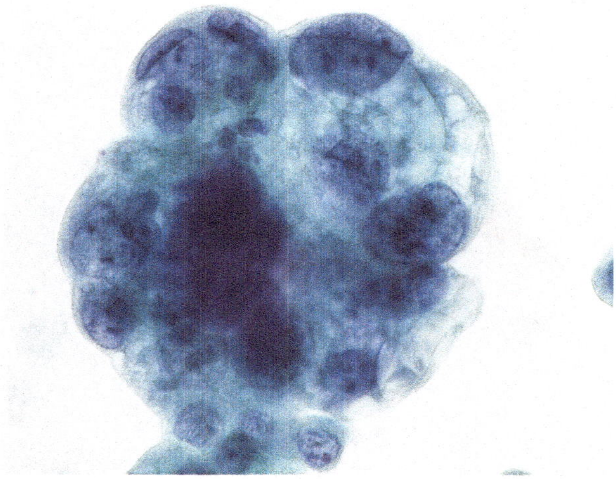

Fig. 6.7 High-grade urothelial carcinoma (HGUC) with cytoplasmic vacuolization reflects glandular differentiation. Nuclear membrane irregularity, hyperchromasia, and coarse chromatin typify HGUC (*Bladder washing, TP, high mag.*)

Definition of HGUC with Glandular Differentiation

Glandular differentiation is defined as the presence of true glandular formation within groups of tumor cells. Glandular cells are intermixed with malignant cells exhibiting classic features of HGUC (Figs. 6.11 and 6.12). Diagnosis of adenocarcinoma of the urinary tract can only be determined by extensive examination of biopsy or cystectomy tissue.

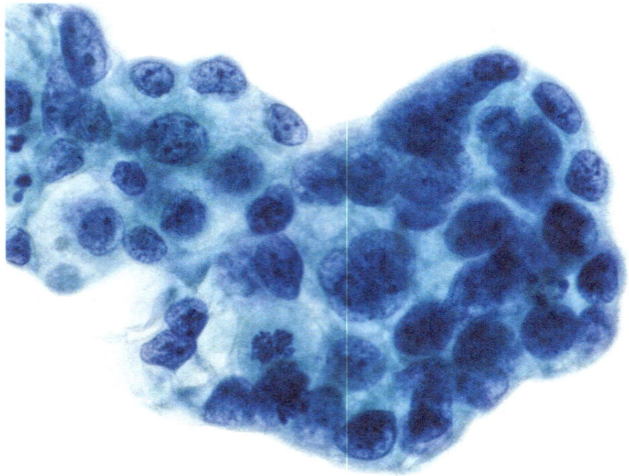

Fig. 6.8 High-grade urothelial carcinoma (HGUC) tumor cells exhibit nuclear hyperchromasia, nuclear membrane irregularity, coarse chromatin, and mitoses. Cytoplasm is frothy and N/C ratios vary, but nuclear features still place the sample in the HGUC category (*Bladder washing, TP, high mag.*)

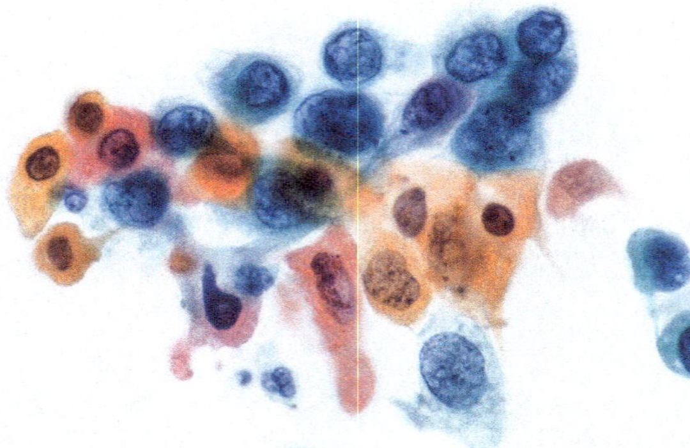

Fig. 6.9 A few cells exhibit classic features of high-grade urothelial carcinoma (HGUC) adjacent to cells of squamous differentiation (*Bladder washing, TP, high mag.*)

Criteria of Malignancy

HGUC is diagnosed on the basis of the following criteria according to The Paris System consensus (see Explanatory Note):

- Cellularity: At least 5–10 abnormal cells
- N/C ratio: 0.7 or greater

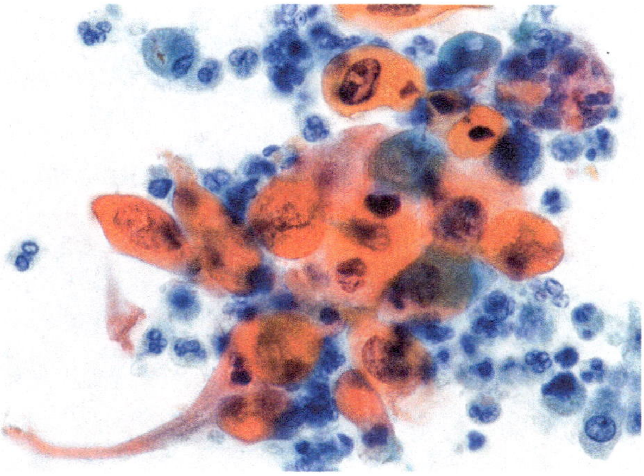

Fig. 6.10 Pronounced keratinization of tumor cells is present in this patient with a history of high-grade urothelial carcinoma (HGUC). The diagnosis of Urothelial Carcinoma vs. Squamous Carcinoma will depend upon the percentage of squamous differentiation once the bladder is removed and completely examined histologically (*Bladder washing, TP, high mag.*)

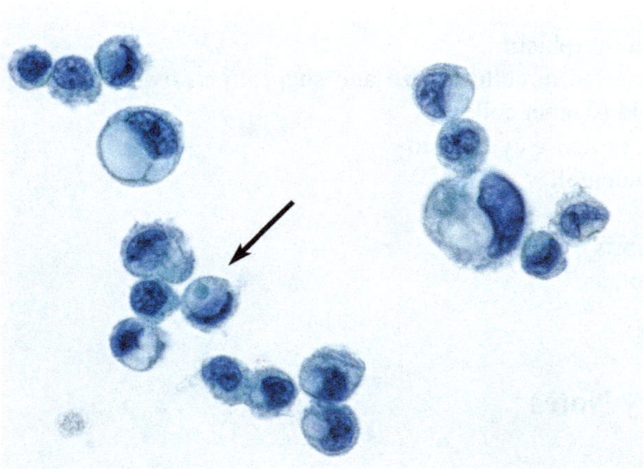

Fig. 6.11 Scattered high-grade urothelial carcinoma (HGUC) tumor cells demonstrate focal glandular differentiation (*Bladder washing, TP, medium mag.*)

- Nucleus: Moderate to severe hyperchromasia
- Nuclear membrane: Markedly irregular
- Chromatin: Coarse/clumped

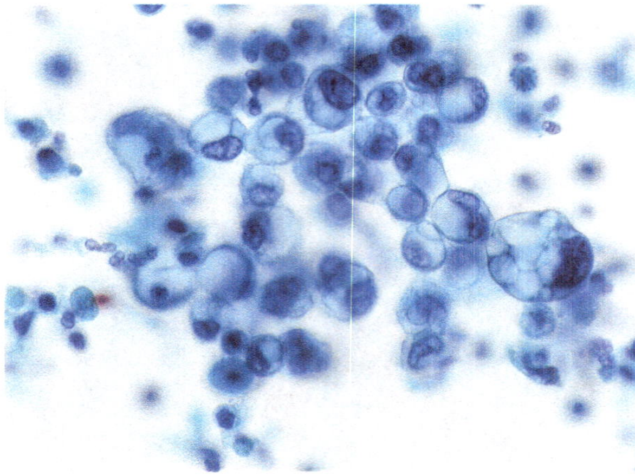

Fig. 6.12 High-grade urothelial carcinoma (HGUC) tumor cells with glandular differentiation are from the same sample as Fig. 6.11 (*Bladder washing, TP, high mag.*)

Other Notable Cytomorphologic Features

- Cellular pleomorphism
- Marked variation in cellular size and shapes, i.e., oval, rounded, elongated, or plasmacytoid (Comet cells)
- Scant, pale, or dense cytoplasm
- Prominent nucleoli
- Mitoses
- Necrotic debris
- Inflammation

Explanatory Notes

Explanatory Note 1: Increased N/C ratio of at least 0.7 is used as a benchmark, in addition to severe hyperchromasia and/or marked nuclear irregularity, for guiding the cytopathologist in identifying malignancy. The majority of HGUC cells will exhibit N/C ratio greater than 0.7, although some cells may show N/C ratio in the range of 0.5–0.7.

Explanatory Note 2: Hyperchromasia is characterized by tumor cells showing a marked density of the nuclear chromatin. Hyperchromasia is moderate to severe in intensity, and should clearly separate the HGUC cells from benign cells present in the sample.

Explanatory Note 3: Prominent nucleoli can be identified in HGUC but may also be present in reactive urothelial cells. Reactive urothelial cells will not exhibit the other criteria of HGUC: hence prominent nucleoli accompanying other criteria of HGUC will be noted in the malignant cells.

Rate of Malignancy

The percentage of urinary cytology cases reported as "positive for malignancy" is relatively low and would be expected to vary based on the clinical and demographic characteristics (risk) of the population, and the practice habits of physicians who are ordering urinary cytology evaluations. Therefore, laboratories may have quite different rates of cases interpreted as "positive for malignancy". It is also noteworthy that patients with cytologic results of "positive for malignancy" and "suspicious for malignancy" are often managed similarly. Thus many studies appropriately combine these two categories when evaluating the diagnostic accuracy of urinary cytology.

In Dr. Papanicolaou's initial publication demonstrating the feasibility of using urinary cytology to detect bladder cancer, 27 of 83 cases, or 33 % were reported as positive for neoplasm [24]. Undoubtedly this cohort of patients was a selected and high-risk population. More contemporary, larger studies from laboratories have reported much lower rates of malignancy that have ranged from 1.7 to 5.8 % of all urinary cytology cases [25–27]. These studies also confirmed that bladder washings and upper urinary tract specimens tend to have a higher percentage of malignant cases as compared to voided urine specimens.

The Paris System working group also made an international outreach attempt to further ascertain the rate of malignancy in various academic and nonacademic practice settings. The data from this study are included in Table 6.1. The cytopathology laboratories contributing these data included both academic and nonacademic practices, and provided data for the year 2013. The rate of malignancy or cases identified as "positive for malignancy" ranged from 1.0 to 6.3 %. In addition, cases that were suspicious for malignancy showed a range of 0.2 to 5.4 %. This again, demonstrates a low number of cases being finalized as equivocal, in most clinical laboratories. The cases that were designated as "Negative for malignancy" ranged from 64.8 to 96.1 %, which demonstrates that the majority of the samples reviewed are benign.

Risk of Malignancy

Studies of the performance of urinary cytology have consistently shown that false positive tests are infrequent when "positive for malignant cells" is considered a diagnostic test. Thus the positive predictive value and specificity of urinary cytology

Table 6.1 The Paris Group outreach survey for rate of malignancy in urinary cytologic specimens in clinical laboratories

Location	Type	Total number	Positive for malignant cells [PFMC] (%)	Suspicious for malignant cells [SFMC] (%)	Atypical NOS (%)	Negative (%)	Washing (%)
Charlotte, NC	Academic/PP	1808	1.0	0.7	3.5	94.8	9.0
New York, NY	Academic	9120	1.0	1.3	4.3	93.4	N/A
Columbia, SC	Academic/PP	841	1.1	1.8	8.2	88.9	N/A
Springfield, IL	PP	1529	1.2	1.8	21.4	75.6	1.4
Denver, CO	Academic	956	1.3	3.7	19.6	75.4	1.0
Worcester, MA	Academic	6853	1.9	1.1	15.9	81.1	1.0
Brunswick, GA	PP	2688	1.9	0.8	20.9	76.4	4.4
St. Louis, MO	Academic	2073	2.0	3.6	15.4	79	N/A
Bangor, ME	PP	3069	2.0	1.2	N/A	96.1	N/A
Montreal, Canada	Academic	6043	2.6	1.9	17.3	78.2	16.1
Longview, TX	PP	722	2.1	0.2	3.1	94.6	20.1
Hammond, IN	PP	734	2.7	1.8	9.7	95.8	N/A
Seattle, WA	PP	3987	3.1	2.6	14.7	79.6	N/A
Maywood, IL	Academic	2005	3.27	1.25	6.09	89.3	74
Nagoya, Japan	PP	4932	3.3	1.2	7.3	88.2	1.0
Kyoto, Japan	Academic	2796	3.5	1.4	2.9	92.1	12.2
Trenton, NJ	PP	81	4.9	2.7	21	71.4	22.2
Toulouse, France	Academic	2380	5.1	0.8	1.8	92.3	N/A
Brunswick, NJ	Academic	1270	6.1	5.4	23.7	64.8	17.4
Atlanta, GA	Academic	1184	6.3	4.5	5.2	83.7	4.0

PP private practice, *N/A* not applicable

designated as "Positive for malignancy" are very high. Studies have reported specificities ranging from 78 to 100 % for positive urine cytology cases, with the majority of them reporting specificities >90 % [19, 25–29]. It should be noted that some of these studies regarded "Suspicious for malignancy" as a positive test. Assessing urinary cytology with immediate histologic follow-up as the gold standard (a common study design) resulted in some true positive cases being misclassified as false positives. The "anticipatory positive" phenomena, i.e., positive urinary cytology with a period of clinically undetectable disease followed by development or discovery of occult urothelial carcinoma, is well known; therefore, some studies with shorter follow-up underestimate the true specificity and positive predictive value of urinary cytology. Because of the high risk of malignancy, a positive urine cytology of HGUC will be followed clinically by cystoscopic examination with biopsies of any lesions detected or suspected as CIS and additional assessment of the upper urothelial tract for clinical disease if necessary.

References

1. Ramakumar S, Bhuiyan J, Besse JA, Roberts SG, Wollan PC, Blute ML, O'Kane DJ. Comparison of screening methods in the detection of bladder cancer. J Urol. 1999;161: 388–94.
2. Karakiewicz PI, Benayoun S, Zippe C, Lüdecke G, Boman H, Sanchez-Carbayo M, et al. Institutional variability in the accuracy of urinary cytology for predicting recurrence of transitional cell carcinoma of the bladder. BJU Int. 2006;97:997–1001.
3. Owens CL, VandenBussche CJ, Burroughs FH, Rosenthal DL. A review of reporting systems and terminology for urine cytology. Cancer Cytopathol. 2013;121:9–14.
4. Papanicolaou GN. Cytology of the urine sediment in neoplasms of the urinary tract. J Urol. 1947;57:375–9.
5. Koss LG, Bartels PH, Sychra JJ, Wied GL. Diagnostic cytologic sample profiles in patients with bladder cancer using TICAS system. Acta Cytol. 1978;22:392–7.
6. Epstein JI, Amin MB, Reuter VR, Mostofi FK. The World Health Organization/International Society of Urological Pathology consensus classification of urothelial (transitional cell) neoplasms of the urinary bladder. Bladder Consensus Conference Committee. Am J Surg Pathol. 1998;22:1435–48.
7. Layfield LJ, Elsheikh TM, Fili A, Nayar R, Shidam V, Papanicolaou Society of Cytopathology. Review of the state of the art and recommendations of the Papanicolaou Society of Cytopathology for urinary cytology procedures and reporting: the Papanicolaou Society of Cytopathology Practice Guidelines Task Force. Diagn Cytopathol. 2004;30:24–30.
8. Li HX, Wang MR, Zhao H, Cao J, Li CL, Pan QJ. Comparison of fluorescence in situ hybridization, nmp22 bladderchek, and urinary liquid-based cytology in the detection of bladder urothelial carcinoma. Diagn Cytopathol. 2013;41:852–7.
9. Yafia FA, Brimob F, Auger M, Aprikian A, Tanguay S, Kassouf W. Is the performance of urinary cytology as high as reported historically? A contemporary analysis in the detection and surveillance of bladder cancer. Urol Oncol. 2014;32:27.e1–e6.
10. Tanaka N, Kikuchi E, Kanao K, Matsumoto K, Shirotake S, Kobayashi H, et al. The predictive value of positive urine cytology for outcomes following radical nephroureterectomy in patients with primary upper tract urothelial carcinoma: a multi-institutional study. Urol Oncol. 2014;32:48.e19–e26.

11. Kobayashi Y, Saika T, Miyaji Y, Saegusa M, Arata R, Akebi N, et al. Preoperative positive urine cytology is a risk factor for subsequent development of bladder cancer after nephroureterectomy in patients with upper urinary tract urothelial carcinoma. World J Urol. 2012;30:271–5.
12. Zieger K, Wolf H, Olsen PR, Hojgaard K. Long-term follow-up of noninvasive bladder tumors (stage Ta): recurrence and progression. BJU Int. 2000;85:824–8.
13. Okajima E, Fujimoto H, Mizutani Y, Kikuchi E, Koga H, Hinotsu S, Cancer Registration Committee of the Japanese Urological Association. Cancer death from non-muscle invasive bladder cancer: report of the Japanese Urological Association of data from the 1999–2001 registry in Japan. Int J Urol. 2010;17:905–12.
14. Koga F, Kobayashi S, Fujii Y, Ishioka J, Yokoyama M, Nakanishi Y, et al. Significance of positive urine cytology on progression and cancer-specific mortality of non-muscle-invasive bladder cancer. Clin Genitourin Cancer. 2014;12:e87–93.
15. Pan CC, Chang YH, Chen KK, Yu HJ, Sun CH, Ho DM. Prognostic Significance of the 2004 WHO/ISUP classification for prediction of recurrence, progression, and cancer-specific mortality of non-muscle-invasive urothelial tumors of the urinary bladder a clinicopathologic study of 1,515 cases. Am J Clin Pathol. 2010;133:788–95.
16. Cheng L, MacLennan GT, Lopez-Beltran A. Histologic grading of urothelial carcinoma: a reappraisal. Human Pathol. 2012;43:2097–108.
17. Bhatia A, Dey P, Kakkar N, Srinivasan R, Nijhawan R. Malignant atypical cell in urine cytology: a diagnostic dilemma. CytoJournal. 2006;3:28.
18. Potts SA, Thomas PA, Cohen MB, Raab SS. Diagnostic accuracy and key cytologic features of high-grade transitional cell carcinoma in the upper urinary tract. Mod Pathol. 1997;10: 657–62.
19. Reid MD, Osunkoya AO, Siddiqui MT, Looney SW. Accuracy of grading of urothelial carcinoma on urine cytology: an analysis of interobserver and intraobserver agreement. Int J Clin Exp Pathol. 2012;5:882–91.
20. Sauter G, Algaba F, Amin MB, Busch C, Cheville J, Gasser T, et al. Non-invasive urothelial neoplasias: WHO classification of noninvasive papillary urothelial tumors. In: Eble JN, Sauter G, Epstein JI, Sesterhenn IA, editors. World Health Organization classification of tumors. Pathology and genetics of tumors of the urinary system and male genital organs. Lyon: IARCC; 2004. p. 110.
21. Reuter VE. The pathology of bladder cancer: a review of its diverse morphology. Urology. 2006;67(3 Suppl 1):11–7; discussion 17–8.
22. Eble JN, Young RH. Carcinoma of the urinary bladder: a review of its diverse morphology. Semin Diagn Pathol. 1997;14:98–108.
23. Lopez-Beltran A, Cheng L. Histologic variants of urothelial carcinoma: a differential diagnosis and clinical implications. Hum Pathol. 2006;37:1371–88.
24. Papanicolaou GN, Marshall VF. Urine sediment smears as a diagnostic procedure in cancers of the urinary tract. Science. 1945;101:519–20.
25. Raab SS, Grzybicki DM, Vrbin CM, Geisinger KR. Urine cytology discrepancies: frequency, causes, and outcomes. Am J Clin Pathol. 2007;127:946–53.
26. Sternberg I, Rona R, Olsfanger S, Lew S, Leibovitch I. The clinical significance of class III (suspicious) urine cytology. Cytopathology. 2011;22:329–33.
27. Rosenthal DL, VandenBussche CJ, Burroughs FH, Sathiyamoorthy S, Guan H, Owens C. The Johns Hopkins Hospital template for urologic cytology samples: part I—creating the template. Cancer Cytopathol. 2013;121:15–20.
28. Ton Nu TN, Kassouf W, Ahmadi-Kaliji B, Charbonneau M, Auger M, Brimo F. The value of the "suspicious for urothelial carcinoma" cytology category: a correlative study of 4 years including 337 patients. Cancer Cytopathol. 2014;22:796–803.
29. Ubago JM, Mehta V, Wojcik EM, Barkan GA. Evaluation of atypical urine cytology progression to malignancy. Cancer Cytopathol. 2013;121:387–91.

Chapter 7
Low-Grade Urothelial Neoplasia (LGUN)

Eva M. Wojcik, Tatjana Antic, Ashish Chandra, Michael B. Cohen, Zulfia McCroskey, Jae Y. Ro, and Taizo Shiraish

Background

Through the years there have been a number of classification schemes that have tried to categorize urinary bladder cancers according to the morphologic appearances. These attempts were proposed to more accurately predict their biology, i.e., recurrence, progression, and the development of new tumors. In 1998 the World Health Organization (WHO) in association with the International Society of Urological Pathology (ISUP) developed a revised system for noninvasive papillary and flat urothelial lesions. It was adopted in 2004 for the WHO's most recent classification "Pathology of the Urinary System and Male Genital Organs." It distinguishes a flat dysplasia from carcinoma in situ (CIS) and categorizes papillary urothelial neoplasms into four groups (Table 7.1): urothelial papilloma, papillary urothelial neoplasm of low malignant potential (PUNLMP), low-grade papillary urothelial carcinoma (LGPUC), and high-grade papillary urothelial carcinoma (HGPUC). Although this classification has gained acceptance, the published comparisons have not clearly confirmed that the 2004 WHO/ISUP classification has better reproducibility than the 1973 WHO classification [1–3]. In addition, despite well-defined criteria, there is a significant variability among pathologists with general agreement in grading, ranging between 50 and 60 % [4–7]. It is further recognized that there is a tendency to underdiagnose HGUC at a rate of 15 % on histology [6].

The authors of the 2004 WHO/ISUP classification clearly stated that their work was still in progress [8]. They also mentioned that, as a group of genetically stable tumors, the noninvasive LGPUCs most likely do not deserve to be designated as cancers. Noninvasive LGPUC remains an anomaly in cancer reporting. No other cancers in the human body (unless it is carcinoma in situ) are called carcinoma by a pathologist in the absence of invasion or are reported as such. Perhaps, it is time for the WHO, ISUP, and other interested groups, e.g., urologists, to address this anomalous terminology.

D.L. Rosenthal et al. (eds.), *The Paris System for Reporting Urinary Cytology*,
DOI 10.1007/978-3-319-22864-8_7

Table 7.1 Grading of non-invasive urothelial neoplasms

WHO 1973 classification		2004 WHO/ISUP classification
Urothelial papilloma		Urothelial papilloma
Grade 1	→ ↘	Papillary urothelial neoplasm of low malignant potential
Grade 2	→ ↘	Low grade papillary urothelial carcinoma
Grade 3	→	High grade papillary urothelial carcinoma
Carcinoma in situ		Carcinoma in situ

ISUP International Society of Urologic Pathologists

Definitions

Histologic Definition of Urothelial Papilloma [8]

Urothelial papilloma is defined as a discrete delicate papillary growth with a central fibrovascular core lined by urothelium indistinguishable from that of the normal urothelium (usually not more than seven cells thick).

Histologic Definition of Papillary Urothelial Neoplasm of Low Malignant Potential [8]

PUNLMP is defined as a papillary urothelial tumor that resembles urothelial papilloma with delicate papillae, but has increased cellular thickness of normal-appearing urothelium, usually more than seven cells thick. Cytologically, there is absent to minimal variation in nuclear atypia, although the nuclei might be slightly enlarged and elongated compared to normal.

Histologic Definition of Low-Grade Papillary Urothelial Carcinoma [8]

LGPUCs are usually small, confined to the urothelium without stromal invasion, and are treated by local excision [3]. They are characterized by thin papillary fronds that show frequent branching, minimal fusion, orderly appearance, and mild variations in architectural features. In contrast to urothelial papilloma or PUNLMP, there is mild but recognizable nuclear atypia such as variations in polarity, size, shape, nuclear border, and chromatin pattern.

Histologic Definition of Urothelial Dysplasia: Flat Low-Grade Intraurothelial Neoplasia [8]

Flat low-grade intraurothelial neoplasia is a flat lesion showing minimal architectural disorganization and some cytologic atypia that is not severe enough to qualify for the diagnosis of CIS. These lesions show variable and often visible loss of polarity. The nuclei of the cells may have irregular nuclear borders, slightly altered chromatin pattern, inconspicuous nucleoli, and rare mitoses.

Cytologic Definition of Low-Grade Urothelial Neoplasia

In keeping with the 2004 WHO/ISUP terminology, low-grade urothelial neoplasia (LGUN) is regarded as a combined cytologic term for low-grade papillary urothelial neoplasms (LGPUN) (which includes urothelial papilloma, PUNLMP and LGPUC) and flat, low-grade intraurothelial neoplasia. We support the view, which represents the current consensus in the field of cytopathology that we should not try to differentiate these entities in urinary tract cytologic specimens [9–11]. Most importantly, it is crucial to separate these entities from HGUC and CIS, which are discussed in Chap. 6. We also recognize that cytologic distinction between low-grade lesions and normal urothelium is extremely difficult. Therefore the only circumstances in which we can make a definitive diagnosis are described below.

Cytologic Criteria of LGUN (Regardless of the Specimen Type: Voided or Instrumented)

Three-dimensional cellular papillary clusters (defined as clusters of cells with nuclear overlapping, forming "papillae") with fibrovascular cores including capillaries (Figs. 7.1, 7.2, and 7.3a). Only in the presence of this feature is the definitive cytologic diagnosis of LGUN possible [9].

In the presence of the features listed below, the cytologic diagnosis of LGUN may be considered, particularly in correlation with cystoscopic or biopsy findings [12]; however, these cases should be categorized as "Negative for High-Grade Urothelial Carcinoma (NHGUC)" (Figs. 7.4, 7.5, 7.6, and 7.7):

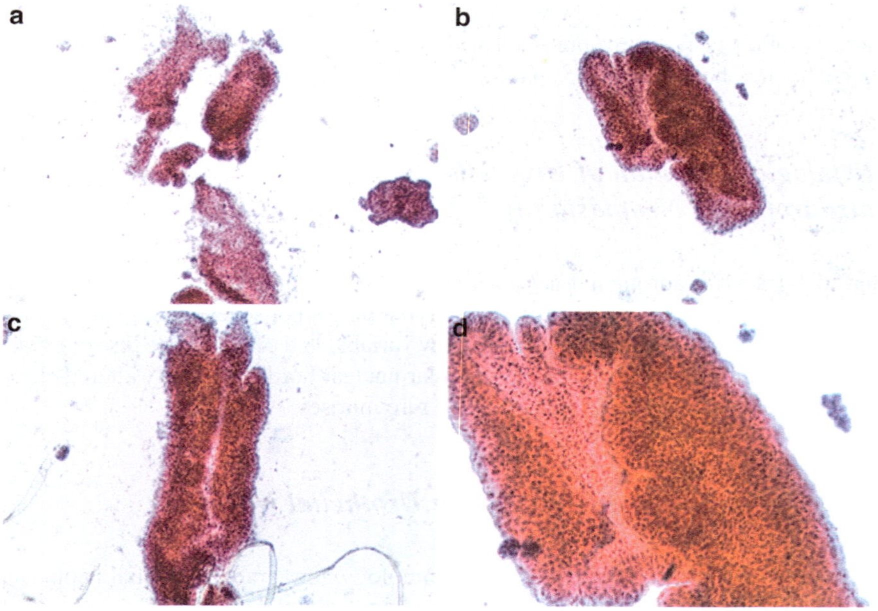

Fig. 7.1 Positive for LGUN (composite). (**a**) Highly cellular specimen composed of numerous tissue fragments. (**b**)–(**d**) Some fragments show three-dimensional papillary configuration. Fibrovascular cores are appreciated in the center of papillary structures (*Renal pelvic washing, CS,* (**a**)–(**c**) *low mag.* (**d**) *medium mag.*)

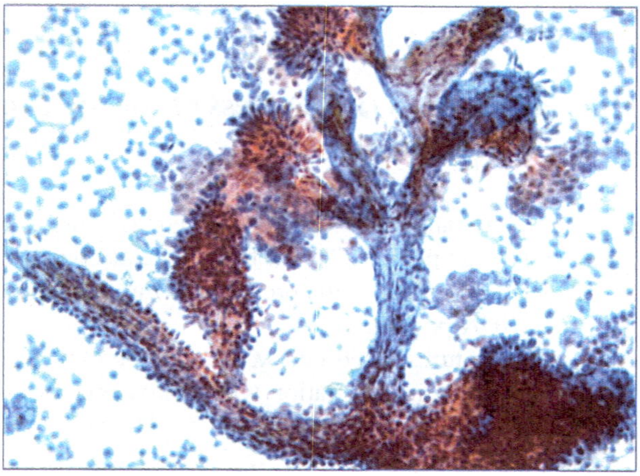

Fig. 7.2 Positive for LGUN. Three-dimensional papillary structures have central cores. Notice mild cytologic atypia and disorganization of cells forming papillae. Photo courtesy of David Wilbur (*Renal pelvic washing, CS, medium mag.*)

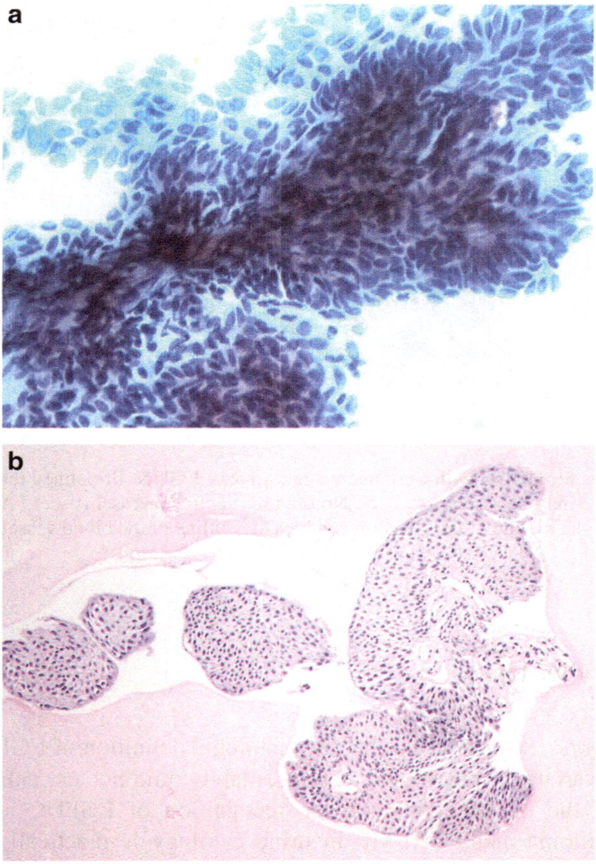

Fig. 7.3 Positive for LGUN. (**a**) Three-dimensional cluster of cells with nuclear overlapping, forming papillae. There is a thin capillary vessel running through the center of the cluster (*Washing, TP, low mag.*). (**b**) Positive for LGUN. Occasionally, if there is enough material left in a container, a cell block may be helpful to visualize fibrovascular cores (*Washing, Cell block, H&E stain, low mag.*)

- Three-dimensional cellular clusters *without* fibrovascular cores (Fig. 7.5a)
- Increased numbers of monotonous single (non-umbrella) cells (Fig. 7.5b)

The following features, although previously reported as characteristic for LGPUC [13–15], may also be associated with high-grade urothelial carcinoma (HGUC) [16]. In the absence of other HGUC characteristics, these cytomorphologic features may suggest a LGUN lesion (see Fig. 7.4). Again, these cases should be categorized as NHGUC:

- Cytoplasmic homogeneity (Fig. 7.6)
- Nuclear border irregularity (Fig. 7.7)
- Increased nuclear/cytoplasmic ratio

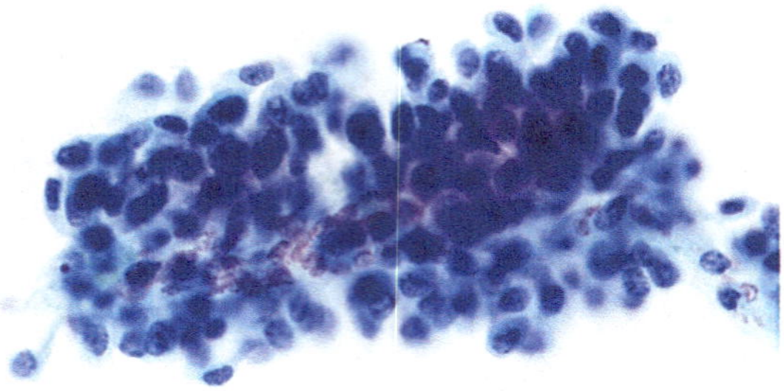

Fig. 7.4 Negative for HGUC with a comment suggestive of LGUN. Ill-defined three-dimensional papillary structure may represent a LGUN. No obvious capillary vessel is seen. Accumulation of red blood cells in the middle of the cluster resembles the outline of the blood vessel wall (*Washing, TP, medium mag.*)

Explanatory Notes

Explanatory Note 1. Considering that the histologic definition of LGPUC includes only minimal variation in cytologic features, mainly mild nuclear enlargement and irregularity of the nuclear contours, the recognition of LGPUC separate from urothelial papilloma and PUNLMP in urine cytology is practically impossible. Relatively few studies have been done on cytopathology specimens to define the cytologic features of LGPUC in urine specimens. Although earlier reports [13, 14, 17] listed three key morphologic features based on which the diagnosis of LGPUC could be made (nuclear enlargement, slight nuclear contour irregularity, and cytoplasmic homogeneity), the reported sensitivity and interobserver agreement for cytologic diagnosis of LGPUC remained low [9, 18, 19]. Those studies were based on highly selected populations of only lower urinary tract specimens, with a very high index of suspicion, retrospective reviews of the morphologic features and long-term follow-up after the initial positive cytologic diagnosis [13, 15]. Most importantly, in some of those studies, grade-2 tumors (transitional cell carcinoma, grade 2) were included in the group of low-grade tumors. Since the introduction of the 2004 WHO/ISUP classification, there has been a significant shift in grading of urothelial neoplasms. Tumors previously classified as grade 2 are now more often categorized as high-grade [5, 6, 20].

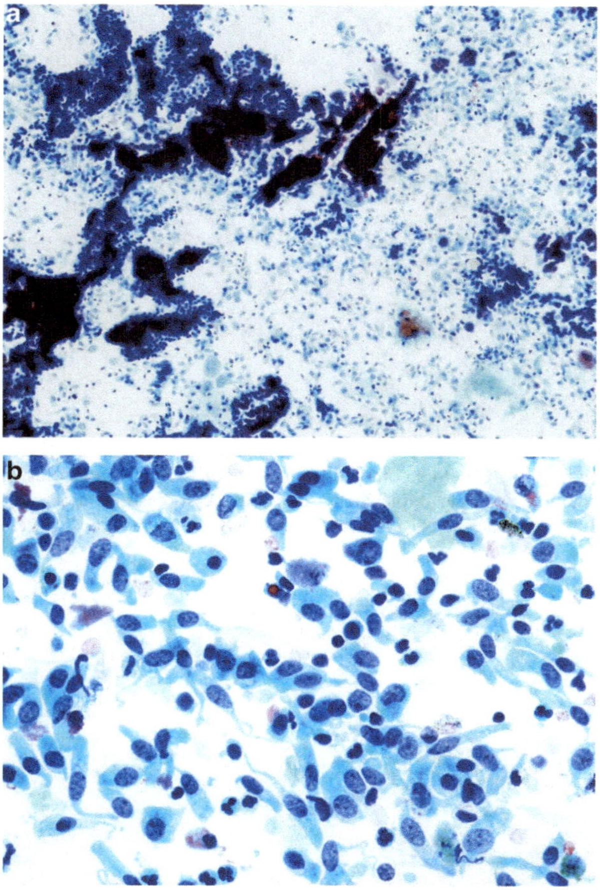

Fig. 7.5 Negative for HGUC with a comment suggestive of LGUN. (**a**) Highly cellular specimen with numerous three-dimensional tissue fragments. No fibrovascular cores were found (*Washing, TP, low mag.*). (**b**) Negative for HGUC with a comment suggestive of LGUN. Abundant single uniform cells in a shape of "cercaria" with elongated tails and eccentrically located nuclei (*Washing, TP, high mag.*)

Explanatory Note 2. Similar to earlier reports [11, 18], in a recent study [21] the majority of the features described previously as diagnostic for LGPUC were observed almost equally in patients with or without biopsy-proven LGPUC, regardless of whether the specimens were from the upper or the lower urinary tract. Specifically, mild nuclear membrane irregularity was present in 48 % of LGPUC and 47.2 % of negative controls ($p=0.93$); mild nuclear enlargement was observed in 42.9 % of LGPUC patients and 49.1 % negative controls ($p=0.26$). Although homogeneous cytoplasm and three-dimensional papillary structures with

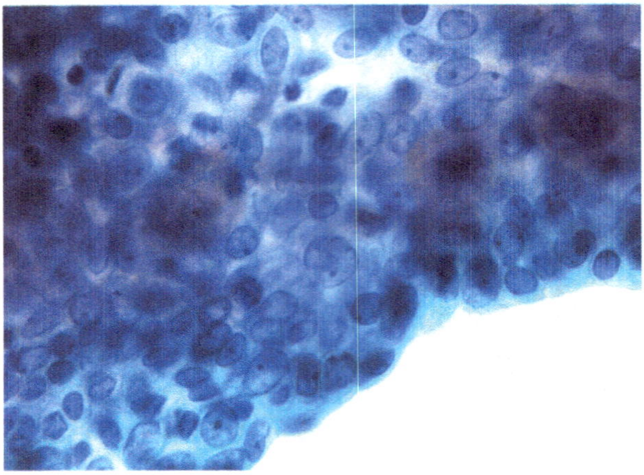

Fig. 7.6 Negative for HGUC with a comment suggestive of LGUN. A cell cluster is composed of urothelial cells with mild cytologic atypia, increased nuclear/cytoplasmic ratios, nuclear overlapping, anisocytosis, slightly irregular nuclear membranes, and dense cytoplasm (*Washing, TP, high mag.*)

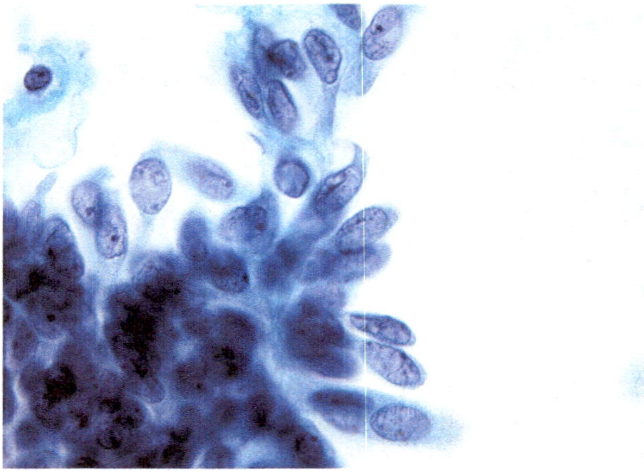

Fig. 7.7 Negative for HGUC with a comment suggestive of LGUN. A cell cluster composed of urothelial cells with mild cytologic atypia demonstrates increased nuclear/cytoplasmic ratios, oval nuclei with occasional grooves and slightly irregular nuclear borders (*Washing, TP, high mag.*)

fibrovascular cores were found only in LGPUC, there were many that did not show these features. Hence, these criteria were not statistically significant in this study.

According to most cytologists, the only time a definitive diagnosis of LGPUC can be rendered in instrumented urine is when well-defined fibrovascular cores (with capillaries) are present [9]; this finding, however, is exceedingly rare.

Explanatory Note 3. Occasionally the specimen will be very cellular and composed of very uniform, mostly singly arranged cells. In these cases umbrella cells are usually lacking or they are rare (see Fig. 7.5a). Individual cells have minimal cytologic atypia (see Fig. 7.5b). In these instrumented specimens it may be possible to suggest a LGPUN; however, in these cases tumors are usually large and are easily visualized during cystoscopy. These cases should still be categorized as "Negative for HGUC" with an optional comment that LGUN is considered.

Explanatory Note 4. The features of flat low-grade intraurothelial dysplasia have been defined by histopathologists [22, 23]. Since Murphy's seminal work in 1984 [13], followed by Dean et al., in 1987 [24], where the authors described cytomorphologic features of urothelial dysplasia in urine specimens, other cytopathologists have not been able to obtain similar results [25]. Moreover, many cytologic reporting templates that have been proposed since that time [26] omitted urothelial dysplasia from their diagnoses. Indeed, even among histopathologists, the reproducibility rate of low-grade flat urothelial dysplasia diagnosis is low [27, 28]. From the clinical viewpoint, most of the urothelial dysplasias occur as secondary lesions or simultaneously with other neoplasms in the bladder [27] and they rarely progress into invasive carcinoma [8].

The cytologic atypia present in individual cells of LGPUNs or flat urothelial dysplasia specimens can be very subtle and not well recognized by cytologists. The cytologic and histologic features of LGPUNs can overlap to some degree as well. We, therefore, recommend that "low-grade urothelial neoplasia" (LGUN) is a better cytologic term that encompasses low-grade papillary neoplasms (urothelial papilloma, PUNLMP, and LGPUC) and flat low-grade urothelial dysplasia.

In daily practice a cytologist should correlate the results of urine cytology with results of cystoscopy and bladder biopsies whenever available. This information should be clearly stated in the report as a note following the diagnosis.

Rate of Recurrence and Risk of Progression

LGPUNs have only few cytogenetic abnormalities, most often a FGFR3 mutation [29], suggesting that these tumors are genetically stable neoplasms [8]. According to the 2004 WHO/ISUP histologic classification, the recurrence rate is 8 % for urothelial papillomas, 35–47 % for PUNLMP, and 48–71 % for LGPUC. These numbers are based on a limited number of studies and it has been reported that progression may be much lower: 0 % for papillomas [30], 3.6 % for PUNLMP [31], and 5–25 % for LGPUC [6, 8, 32]. The relatively high progression rate of LGPUC into HGPUC in some studies can be explained by sampling errors, the tendency to undergrade urothelial carcinomas, as well as grading tumors based on the dominant neoplasm and not the highest-grade pattern [6].

True progression rate of flat urothelial dysplasia is unknown due to lack of information about its true incidence [8]. Some authors reported 15–19 % of progression into CIS, papillary urothelial carcinoma, and HGUC [33, 34].

Due to the aforementioned difficulties in readily identifying low-grade lesions, reflex ancillary testing in the cytology laboratory may be of value. In some cases, where there is material in a container, a cell block preparation [35] would lead to a definitive diagnosis (see Fig. 7.3). Ancillary techniques are discussed under the relevant section (see Chap. 9).

References

1. Babjuk M, Burger M, Zigeuner R, Shariat SF, van Rhijn BW, Comperat E, et al. EAU guidelines on non-muscle-invasive urothelial carcinoma of the bladder: update 2013. Eur Urol. 2013;64:639–53.
2. Curry JL, Wojcik EM. The effects of the current World Health Organization/International Society of Urologic Pathologists bladder neoplasm classification system on urine cytology results. Cancer. 2002;96:140–5.
3. Epstein JI. The new World Health Organization/International Society of Urological Pathology (WHO/ISUP) classification for TA, T1 bladder tumors: is it an improvement? Crit Rev Oncol Hematol. 2003;47:83–9.
4. May M, Brookman-Amissah S, Roigas J, Hartmann A, Störkel S, Kristiansen G, et al. Prognostic accuracy of individual uropathologists in noninvasive urinary bladder carcinoma: a multicentre study comparing the 1973 and 2004 World Health Organisation classifications. Eur Urol. 2010;57:850–8.
5. van Rhijn BW, van Leenders GJ, Ooms BC, Kirkels WJ, Zlotta AR, Boevé ER, et al. The pathologist's mean grade is constant and individualizes the prognostic value of bladder cancer grading. Eur Urol. 2010;57:1052–7.
6. Miyamoto H, Brimo F, Schultz L, Ye H, Miller JS, Fajardo DA, et al. Low-grade papillary urothelial carcinoma of the urinary bladder: a clinicopathologic analysis of a post-World Health Organization/International Society of Urological Pathology classification cohort from a single academic center. Arch Pathol Lab Med. 2010;134:1160–3.
7. Tuna B, Yorukoglu K, Duzcan E, Sen S, Nese N, Sarsik B, et al. Histologic grading of urothelial papillary neoplasms: impact of combined grading (two-numbered grading system) on reproducibility. Virchows Arch. 2011;458:659–64.
8. Sauter G, Algaba F, Amin MB, Busch C, Cheville J, Gasser T, et al. Noninvasive urothelial neoplasias. In: Eble JN, Sauter G, Epstein JI, Sesterhenn IA, editors. World Health Organization classification of tumours. Pathology and genetics of tumors of the urinary system and male genital organs. Lyon: IARCC; 2004. p. 110–23.
9. Renshaw AA, Nappi D, Weinberg DS. Cytology of grade 1 papillary transitional cell carcinoma. A comparison of cytologic, architectural and morphometric criteria in cystoscopically obtained urine. Acta Cytol. 1996;40:676–82.
10. Renshaw AA. Compassionate conservatism in urinary cytology. Diagn Cytopathol. 2000;22:137–8.
11. Layfield LJ, Elsheikh TM, Fili A, Nayar R, Shidham V, Papanicolaou Society of Cytopathology. Review of the state of the art and recommendations of the Papanicolaou Society of Cytopathology for urinary cytology procedures and reporting: the Papanicolaou Society of Cytopathology Practice Guidelines Task Force. Diagn Cytopathol. 2004;30:24–30.
12. Mai KT, Ball CG, Kos Z, Belanger EC, Islam S, Sekhon H. Three-dimensional cell groups with disordered nuclei and cellular discohesion (3DDD) are associated with high sensitivity

and specificity for cystoscopic urine cytopathological diagnosis of low-grade urothelial neoplasia. Diagn Cytopathol. 2014;42:555–63.
13. Murphy WM, Soloway MS, Jukkola AF, Crabtree WN, Ford KS. Urinary cytology and bladder cancer. The cellular features of transitional cell neoplasms. Cancer. 1984;53:1555–65.
14. Raab SS, Lenel JC, Cohen MB. Low grade transitional cell carcinoma of the bladder. Cytologic diagnosis by key features as identified by logistic regression analysis. Cancer. 1994;74:1621–6.
15. Raab SS, Slagel DD, Jensen CS, Teague MW, Savell VH, Ozkutlu D, et al. Low-grade transitional cell carcinoma of the urinary bladder: application of select cytologic criteria to improve diagnostic accuracy [corrected]. Mod Pathol. 1996;9:225–32.
16. Brimo F, Vollmer RT, Case B, Aprikian A, Kassouf W, Auger M. Accuracy of urine cytology and the significance of an atypical category. Am J Clin Pathol. 2009;132:785–93.
17. Hughes JH, Raab SS, Cohen MB. The cytologic diagnosis of low-grade transitional cell carcinoma. Am J Clin Pathol. 2000;114(Suppl):S59–67.
18. Reid MD, Osunkoya AO, Siddiqui MT, Looney SW. Accuracy of grading of urothelial carcinoma on urine cytology: an analysis of interobserver and intraobserver agreement. Int J Clin Exp Pathol. 2012;5:882–91.
19. Renshaw AA. Subclassifying atypical urinary cytology specimens. Cancer. 2000;90:222–9.
20. MacLennan GT, Kirkali Z, Cheng L. Histologic grading of noninvasive papillary urothelial neoplasms. Eur Urol. 2007;51:889–97. discussion 97-8.
21. McCroskey Z, Kliethermes S, Bahar B, Barkan GA, Pambuccian SE, Wojcik EM. Is a consistent cytologic diagnosis of low-grade urothelial carcinoma in instrumented urinary tract cytologic specimens possible? A comparison between cytomorphologic features of low-grade urothelial carcinoma and non-neoplastic changes shows extensive overlap, making a reliable diagnosis impossible. J Am Soc Cytopathol. 2014;4:90–7.
22. Amin MB, Murphy WM, Reuter VE, Ro JY, Ayala AG, Weiss MA, et al. A symposium on controversies in the pathology of transitional cell carcinomas of the urinary bladder. Part I. Anat Pathol. 1996;1:1–39.
23. Amin MB, McKenney JK. An approach to the diagnosis of flat intraepithelial lesions of the urinary bladder using the World Health Organization/ International Society of Urological Pathology consensus classification system. Adv Anat Pathol. 2002;9:222–32.
24. Dean PJ, Murphy WM. Carcinoma in situ and dysplasia of the bladder urothelium. World J Urol. 1987;5:103–7.
25. Ooms EC, Veldhuizen RW. Cytological criteria and diagnostic terminology in urinary cytology. Cytopathology. 1993;4:51–4.
26. Owens CL, VandenBussche CJ, Burroughs FH, Rosenthal DL. A review of reporting systems and terminology for urine cytology. Cancer Cytopathol. 2013;121:9–14.
27. Lopez-Beltran A, Montironi R, Vidal A, Scarpelli M, Cheng L. Urothelial dysplasia of the bladder: diagnostic features and clinical significance. Anal Quant Cytopathol Histpathol. 2013;35:121–9.
28. Amin MB, Trpkov K, Lopez-Beltran A, Grignon D, Members of the ISUP Immunohistochemistry in Diagnostic Urologic Pathology Group. Best practices recommendations in the application of immunohistochemistry in the bladder lesions: report from the International Society of Urologic Pathology consensus conference. Am J Surg Pathol. 2014;38:e20–34.
29. van Rhijn BW, Montironi R, Zwarthoff EC, Jöbsis AC, van der Kwast TH. Frequent FGFR3 mutations in urothelial papilloma. J Pathol. 2002;198:245–51.
30. McKenney JK, Amin MB, Young RH. Urothelial (transitional cell) papilloma of the urinary bladder: a clinicopathologic study of 26 cases. Mod Pathol. 2003;16:623–9.
31. Cheng L, Zhang S, MacLennan GT, Williamson SR, Lopez-Beltran A, Montironi R. Bladder cancer: translating molecular genetic insights into clinical practice. Hum Pathol. 2011;42:455–81.
32. Jackson J, Barkan GA, Kapur U, Wojcik EM. Cytologic and cystoscopic predictors of recurrence and progression in patients with low-grade urothelial carcinoma. Cancer Cytopathol. 2013;121:398–402.

33. Cheng L, Cheville JC, Neumann RM, Bostwick DG. Natural history of urothelial dysplasia of the bladder. Am J Surg Pathol. 1999;23:443–7.
34. Zuk RJ, Rogers HS, Martin JE, Baithun SI. Clinicopathological importance of primary dysplasia of bladder. J Clin Pathol. 1988;41:1277–80.
35. Nathan NA, Narayan E, Smith MM, Horn MJ. Cell block cytology. Improved preparation and its efficacy in diagnostic cytology. Am J Clin Pathol. 2000;114:599–606.

Chapter 8
Other Malignancies Primary and Metastatic and Miscellaneous Lesions

Rana S. Hoda, Stefan E. Pambuccian, Jae Y. Ro, and Sun Hee Sung

Primary Non-Urothelial Tumors

Non-urothelial bladder tumors are uncommon, accounting for less than 5 % of all bladder tumors, and may rarely be detected in urine cytology [1, 2]. Cytological diagnosis of non-urothelial carcinoma (non-UC) and metastasis has rarely been described and frequently poses a diagnostic challenge due to morphological overlap with urothelial carcinoma (UC). Moreover, the cytological distinction between UC with divergent differentiation from pure non-UC may not be possible in cytological samples or in small biopsy specimens, and frequently requires surgical resection. Primary non-UC malignancies pursue an aggressive clinical course and often present at an advanced stage of disease. A multimodal approach using clinical details, imaging results, and pathological diagnosis is vital for a prompt management decision and earlier therapeutic intervention. The overall survival, however, remains poor [3]. Metastasis to the urinary bladder is a rare event and review of the prior primary tumor is necessary to exclude the possibility of an independent primary non-UC [4].

This chapter will review the background, etiology, diagnostic criteria cytology [5, 6], particularly on histological diagnosis and utility of immunocyto- and histochemistry for non-urothelial tumors and metastasis to the bladder.

D.L. Rosenthal et al. (eds.), *The Paris System for Reporting Urinary Cytology*,
DOI 10.1007/978-3-319-22864-8_8

Epithelial Malignancies

Squamous Cell Carcinoma

Background

Squamous cell carcinoma (SqCC) is the second most common malignant neoplasm of the urinary tract, accounting for 2–5 % of all malignancies and 10–20 % of muscle-invasive malignancies of the bladder in the Western world [7]. However, in countries endemic for *Schistosoma hematobium* infection (North Africa and the Middle East), it is responsible for about 25–30 % of all bladder malignancies [8]. Based on etiology and (bilharzial) clinical presentation, SqCC of the urinary tract can be classified as Schistosoma-associated and non-bilharzial. Regardless of their etiology, SqCC of the urinary tract is usually well differentiated (10 %) or moderately differentiated (60 %) and shows abundant keratinization.

Non-bilharzial SqCC of the urinary tract usually occurs in adults with a peak incidence in the seventh decade and typically presents with painless hematuria and irritative symptoms. It is usually associated with conditions leading to urinary stasis with resultant epithelial injury such as spinal cord injury or paraplegic patients and chronic inflammation resulting from smoking, food or bacterial infections, calculi and long-term cyclophosphamide treatment [6, 7].

Bilharzial SqCC of the bladder occurs in the sixth decade in patients with chronic *Schistosoma hematobium* infections (Fig. 8.1a, b). Male to female ratio is 5–6:1 and patients frequently present with pain or a tender palpable mass, and occasionally with necroturia (passage of whitish necrotic tumor fragments) [7].

Definition

SqCC of the urinary tract is a malignant neoplasm that shows exclusively squamous differentiation, without associated urothelial or glandular elements.

Diagnostic Criteria

- Cellular specimen with numerous individual and nests of squamous cells (Figs. 8.2 and 8.3).
- Tumor cells are large, polygonal with keratinized cytoplasm, sharp borders and mildly to markedly atypical hyperchromatic nuclei (Figs. 8.3 and 8.4). Fiber and tadpole cells, squamous pearls and "cell in cell" arrangements may be present.

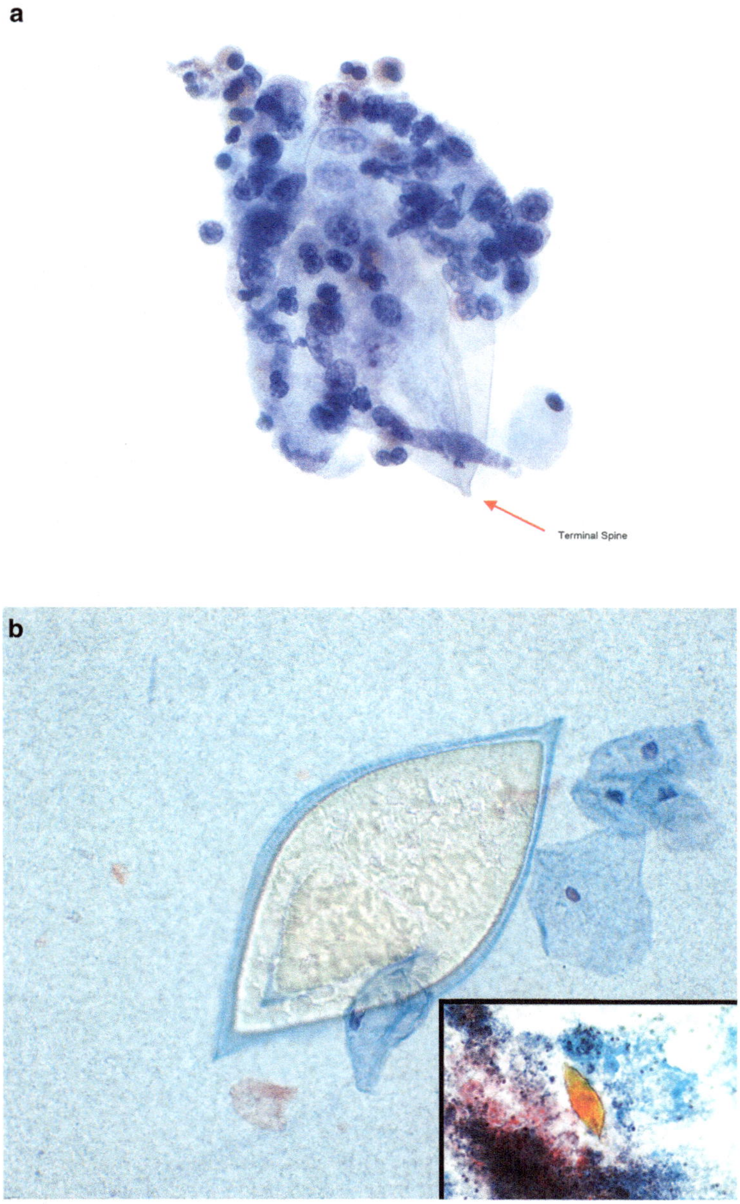

Fig. 8.1 *Schistosoma hematobium* eggs in cytologic preparations. (**a**) *S. hematobium* egg shows an oval structure with a terminal spine (at the end of an oval egg) surrounded by urothelial and inflammatory cells (*Voided urine, TP, high mag.*) (**b**) Well-displayed *S. hematobium* egg in an older filter preparation, note the lancet-shaped terminal and internal egg detail. Preserved squamous cells are present in the background. In the *inset* a *S. hematobium* egg is surrounded by inflammatory cells and debris (*Voided urine; Main Image: Filter Preparation, high mag; Inset: CS, medium mag.*)

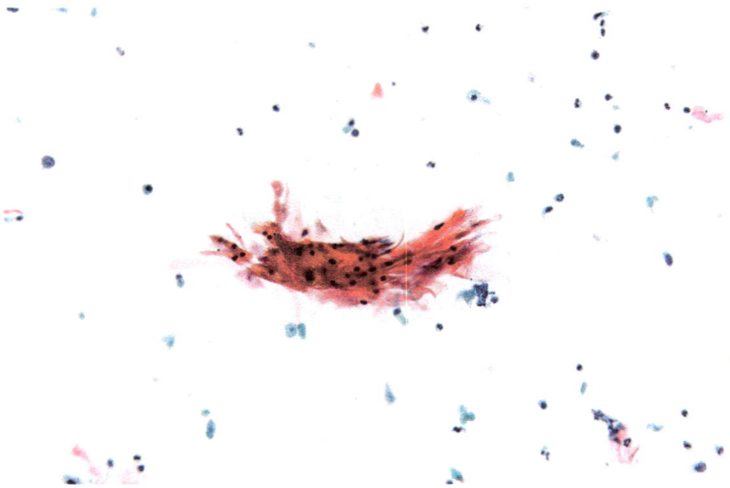

Fig. 8.2 Squamous cell carcinoma (SqCC) of the urinary bladder showing a nest of elongated keratinized "fiber" cells in a background of inflammatory cells and some keratotic debris (*Voided urine, TP, low mag.*)

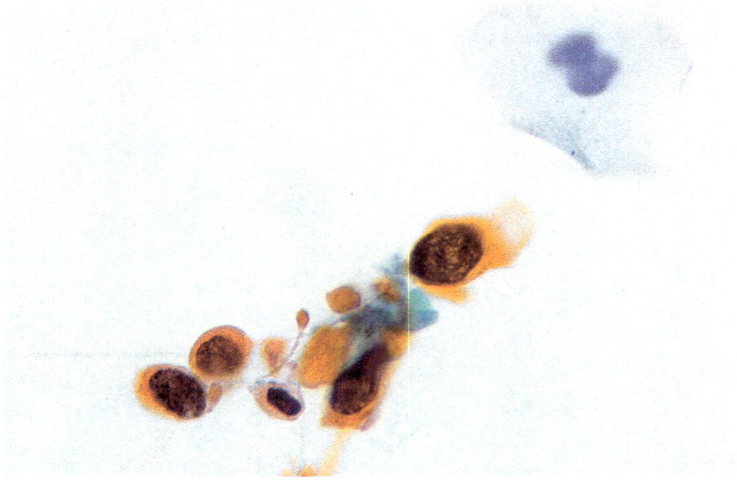

Fig. 8.3 SqCC of urinary bladder with coarse dysplastic nuclear features. Compare the size and staining of the neoplastic cell nuclei to the umbrella cell in the *upper right hand corner* of the image (*Voided urine, TP, medium mag.*)

- Background may show plaques and fragments ("ghost cells") of anucleated squamous cells, small atypical parakeratotic cells, necrosis, red blood cells, and neutrophils (Figs. 8.2 and 8.5).

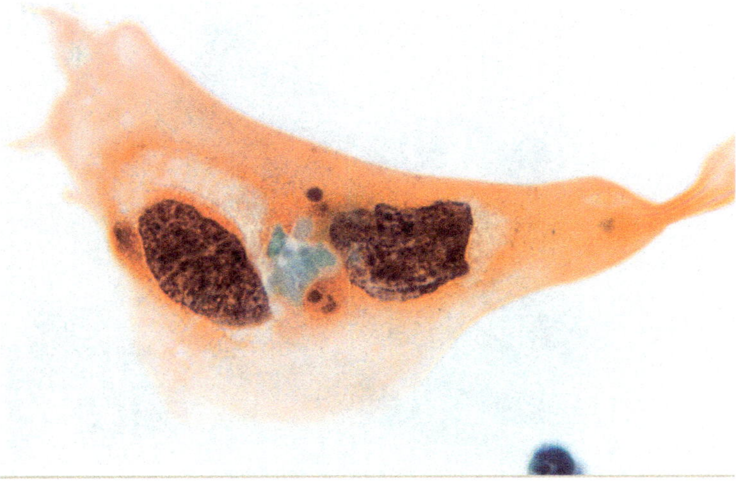

Fig. 8.4 Keratinizing SqCC cells of the urinary bladder display large, polygonal tumor cells with keratinized orangeophilic cytoplasm, sharp borders, and mildly to markedly atypical hyperchromatic nuclei (*Voided urine, TP, high mag.*)

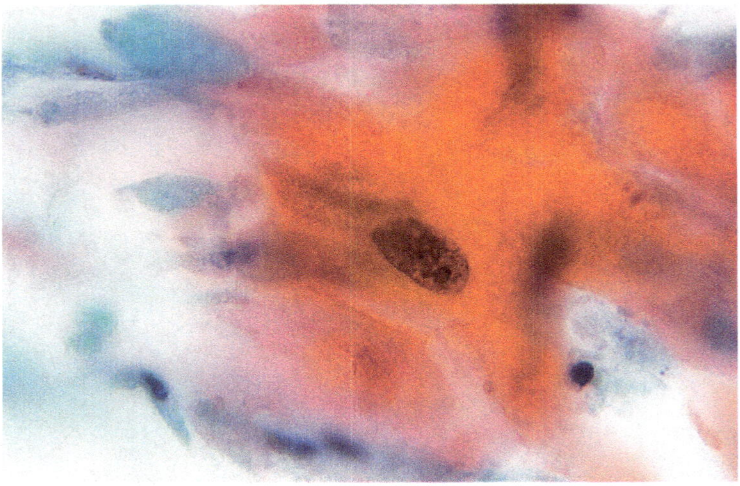

Fig. 8.5 Keratinizing SqCC showing plaque/fragment of anucleated squamous cells ("ghost cells"). Note one nucleated atypical squamous cell in contrast to the degenerating nuclei in the other cells (*Voided urine, TP, medium mag.*)

- Non-keratinizing malignant cell groups with metaplastic appearance may be present (Fig. 8.6).

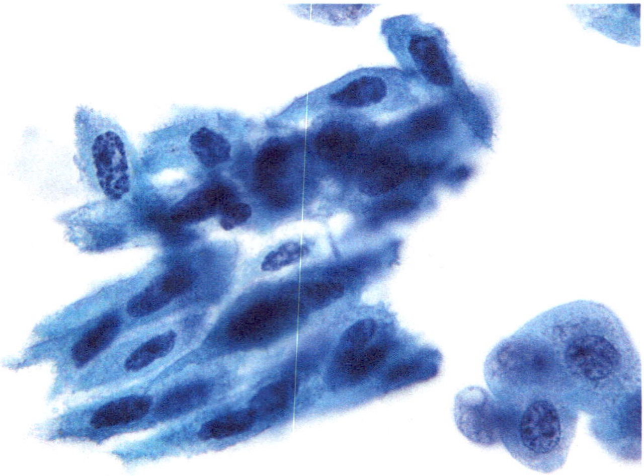

Fig. 8.6 Non-keratinizing SqCC of urinary bladder shows metaplastic type of cells with rigid basophilic cytoplasm and hyperchromatic angulated malignant nuclei (*Voided urine, TP, medium mag.*)

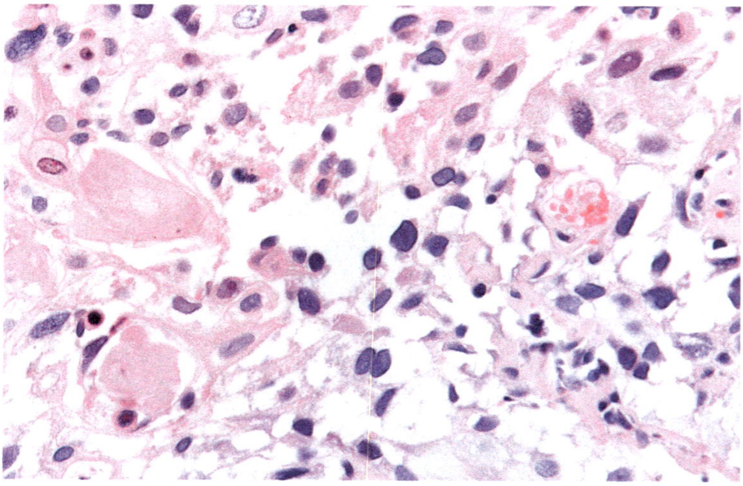

Fig. 8.7 Cell block preparation from the case of keratinizing SqCC shown in Fig. 8.4, has many neoplastic nuclei amid intact and disrupted fragments of keratinized cytoplasm (*H&E, low mag.*)

Liquid-Based Preparations (LBP)

- Show similar morphology as conventional preparations; however, the background is clean so cell details are better preserved [6] (Figs. 8.2, 8.3, and 8.4).
- Cell block section from residual liquid-based specimen can also be prepared (Fig. 8.7).

Explanatory Notes

Explanatory Note 1: Cytologic diagnosis of well-to-moderately differentiated SqCC of the bladder is usually straightforward. Diagnostic difficulties may be encountered for well-differentiated SqCC, which may be difficult to diagnose as malignant, and for poorly differentiated SqCC, which may be difficult to diagnose as squamous.

Explanatory Note 2: In well-differentiated tumors, a careful search may disclose the presence of squamous cells showing nuclear enlargement and hyperchromasia or prominent nuclear membrane irregularity as well as necrotic debris [9]. Occasionally, these tumors are diagnosed as "atypical squamous cells". The differential diagnosis of the latter includes a variety of benign, dysplastic or malignant lesions, including, squamous metaplasia, squamous papilloma, condyloma acuminatum, dysplasia, in situ and invasive SqCC of the bladder as well as contamination from such lesions in the lower female genital tract and UC with divergent squamous differentiation. Since the underlying rate of malignancy associated with "atypical squamous cells" in urine cytology is about 20 % [9], cystoscopy and biopsy may be indicated for these patients. Colposcopy may be required to exclude lower female genital tract origin.

Explanatory Note 3: The diagnosis of SqCC should be accompanied by a disclaimer stating that UC with divergent squamous differentiation cannot be excluded. The diagnosis of pure SqCC should be based on resection specimens. S100P, GATA3, and uroplakin III [10] are, in the order of decreasing sensitivity, immunohistochemical markers that can be used to demonstrate urothelial differentiation.

Adenocarcinoma

Background

Adenocarcinoma (AdCa) is the third most common malignant neoplasm of the urinary tract, accounting for 0.5–2.5 % of all primary bladder malignancies and includes vesical AdCa and urachal AdCa. The latter develops within urachal remnants located in the dome of the bladder and often secondarily involves the bladder [7, 11]. Secondary involvement of the bladder and upper urinary tract by direct extension or metastasis from AdCa from other organs is unusual, but is more common than primary urinary tract AdCa. Risk factors for primary AdCa include bladder exstrophy and cystitis glandularis, intestinal type [7, 12].

Primary bladder and urachal AdCas have similar morphology and can be classified as mucinous, enteric, signet ring cell, mixtures of the above types, and AdCa with no distinctive features, i.e., not otherwise specified (AdCa, NOS). Urachal AdCas are more frequently mucinous ("colloid"), whereas non-urachal AdCa are more frequently AdCa, NOS (Figs. 8.8), and signet ring cell AdCa, which may explain their worse prognosis [13]. While primary bladder AdCas are similar to

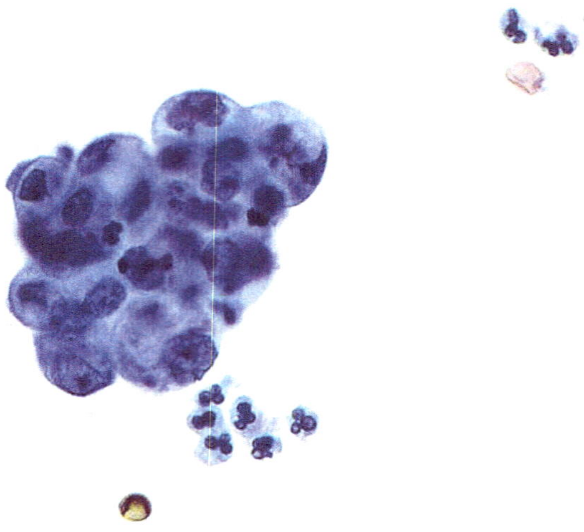

Fig. 8.8 Adenocarcinoma, not otherwise specified (AdCa, NOS) displays a cluster of cells with eccentrically placed irregular nuclei, prominent nucleoli, and finely vacuolated cytoplasm. In an individual fragment it is difficult to determine if the apparent vacuolization is due to glandular secretion or degeneration, but the observation of many such fragments results in a conclusion of glandular differentiation (*Voided urine, TP, high mag.*)

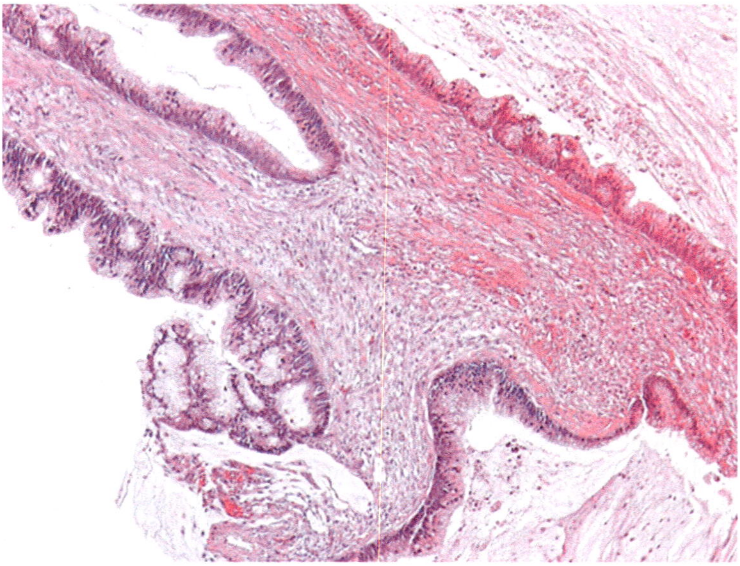

Fig. 8.9 Resected bladder with enteric (colonic) AdCa, exhibiting neoplastic glandular epithelium with tall columnar cells with elongated pencil-shaped nuclei and background mucin (*H&E, low mag.*)

UCs in their age and gender distribution, urachal AdCas occur in a much younger patient population with a median age of around 50 years and have no gender predilection. Clinical symptoms at presentation are hematuria, dysuria, urinary frequency, and rarely mucosuria.

Definition

Primary AdCa of the urinary bladder is a malignant neoplasm derived from metaplastic urothelium showing histologically pure glandular differentiation. Urachal AdCa develops within urachal remnants.

Criteria

- Cellularity of cytologic samples is variable.
- Enteric (colonic-type) AdCa, (Fig. 8.9) show columnar cell clusters and single degenerated cells in a background of necrosis and mucin. Nuclei are large, vesicular or hyperchromatic, with irregular shapes and visible or prominent nucleoli. The cytoplasm may be vacuolated (Fig. 8.10).
- Mucinous (colloid) AdCa show rounded three-dimensional clusters of crowded, rather bland cells with small to moderate amounts of lacy cytoplasm with

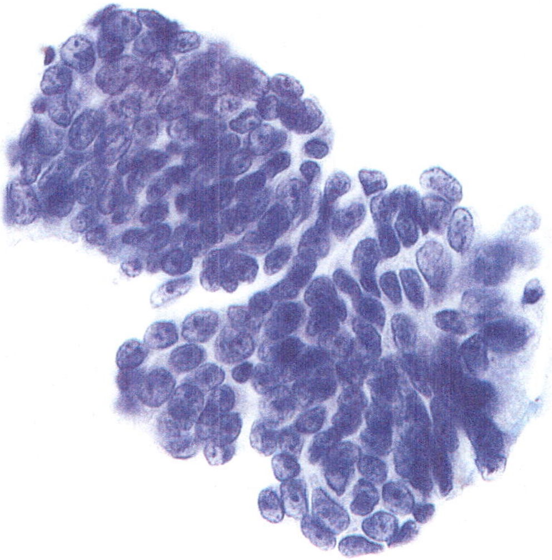

Fig. 8.10 Enteric (colonic-type) AdCa of the urinary bladder demonstrates a cluster of cells. Nuclei are large, columnar to round, irregular, hyperchromatic with thick nuclear membranes and prominent nucleoli. The cytoplasm is scant and vacuolated (*Voided urine, TP, high mag.*)

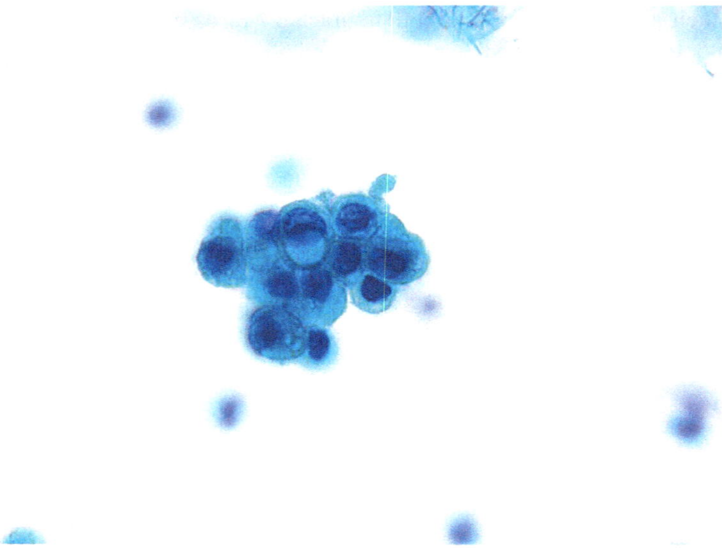

Fig. 8.11 Signet ring cell carcinoma of the urinary bladder displays a cluster of cells with one cell showing a crescent-shaped hyperchromatic nucleus pushed to the periphery of the cell by a large cytoplasmic mucin-containing vacuole (*Voided urine, SP, high mag.*)

occasional mucin vacuoles and medium-sized nuclei with visible nucleoli. Mucin is present in the background.

- Signet ring cell carcinoma displays cells with a large cytoplasmic mucin-containing vacuole that may appear optically clear or finely vacuolated and pushes the crescent-shaped hyperchromatic nucleus to the periphery of the cell (Fig. 8.11).
- Clear cell AdCa has cells with abundant vacuolated cytoplasm and centrally located nuclei that may be present in clusters with hobnail configuration (Fig. 8.12).

Explanatory Notes

Explanatory Note 1: The cytomorphology of AdCa in urinary tract cytology specimens differs according to the type of AdCa, as seen above and usually can be readily diagnosed as malignant [11–13].

Differential diagnosis of well-differentiated primary AdCa of the bladder includes glandular cells from a fistula with the vagina or the gastrointestinal tract, cystitis glandularis, intestinal metaplasia, nephrogenic metaplasia/adenoma, and villous adenoma [7, 14].

Explanatory Note 2: The exclusion of UCs with glandular differentiation may be difficult, and may require the use of immunostains to demonstrate a malignant urothelial component that may be positive (with decreasing frequency) for S100P, p63, and GATA3 [15].

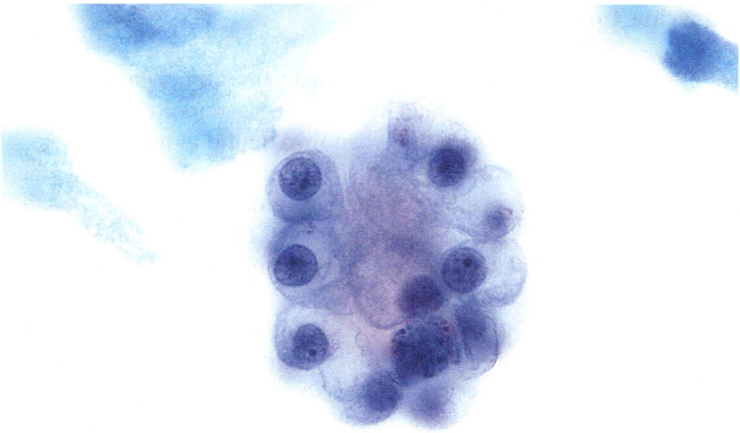

Fig. 8.12 Clear cell AdCa of the urinary bladder is characterized by a cluster of cells with projecting cytoplasm in a "hobnail configuration". The abundant vacuolated cytoplasm and centrally located nuclei with prominent nucleoli complete the features of this subtype of cancer (*Voided urine, TP, high mag.*)

However, the most difficult task is to rule out secondary involvement of the bladder by AdCa from other organs, either by direct extension (colorectal, prostatic, and gynecologic) or by hematogenous metastasis (breast, pancreatic, gastric, and pulmonary). Clinical and imaging correlation and immunostains are most effective in this regard.

Explanatory Note 3: Since most primary AdCas of the bladder have an enteric (colonic) or signet ring cell phenotype, it is important to rule out secondary involvement from a colorectal primary. Although urinary tract AdCas typically express markers of intestinal differentiation (villin, CK20, CEA, and CDX2) and may even harbor KRAS mutations, they lack nuclear beta-catenin expression, which is present in over 80 % of colorectal AdCa, and are frequently positive for CK7 [11]. GATA3 expression may be seen in signet ring cell carcinomas of the bladder, but not in metastatic gastric signet ring cell carcinomas [15]. Clear cell AdCa have to be differentiated from renal cell carcinomas (RCCs) by using renal cell markers, PAX-8, CD10, and CA IX. Prostatic ductal AdCa frequently extends into the bladder or urethra and can show cytological features similar to those of primary urinary tract AdCa from which they can be differentiated due to their PSA immunopositivity [11, 12, 14].

Neuroendocrine Tumors

Two types of neuroendocrine (NE) tumors, with diverse clinicopathological features and outcome, occur in the urinary bladder including carcinoid tumor and neuroendocrine carcinoma (NEC). Both of these can involve the kidney, prostate, and urinary bladder and are morphologically, histochemically, immunohistochemically, and ultrastructurally similar to their counterpart in other organs such as lungs and GI tract. NEC of the urinary bladder with large cell (LCNEC) and small cell NEC morphology are rare entities, accounting for less than 1 % of urinary bladder malignancies. The latter is more common.

The histogenesis of NEC of the bladder remains to be elucidated. Approximately half the reported cases have a mixture with other histologic subtypes in which UC predominates. This supports the most widely accepted view that the NEC of the bladder originates in a pluripotential stem cell that can differentiate into various cell types suggesting a common clonal origin of the NE, urothelial, squamous, or adenocarcinoma component.

Carcinoid. Primary carcinoid tumors of the urinary bladder are exceedingly rare with fewer than 20 pure histologically documented cases reported in the literature. Rarely, carcinoids may be associated with UC. The average age is around 55 years and present with hematuria. The tumor occurs in the trigone and bladder neck as a polypoid or smooth small submucosal nodule and is mostly cured by simple resection. Cytology is similar to carcinoid tumors elsewhere. The prognosis of carcinoid is very favorable; however, it should be distinguished from paraganglioma/pheochromocytoma, NECs, lymphoma, and UC [16].

Small Cell Carcinoma and Large Cell Neuroendocrine Carcinoma

Background

Extrapulmonary small cell carcinoma (SmCC) is rare and can occur at diverse sites including the bladder and accounts for less than 1 % of all urinary bladder carcinomas. Like pulmonary SmCC, it is closely associated with tobacco smoking and is also morphologically and prognostically similar (Fig. 8.13). The most favored histogenesis of the tumor is origin from basally located multipotential stem cells that can differentiate into various cell types. This origin may explain the frequent (more than 50 % of cases) association of SmCC with other carcinomatous components, such as UC, SqCC, AdCa, sarcomatoid carcinoma, or mixtures of these components. Tumors with pure or mixed histologic patterns are classified as SmCC rather than UC, SqCC, or AdCa with NE differentiation [17]. Clinical and other demographic features as well as gross appearance of SmCC are similar to those seen in patients with conventional UC of the bladder.

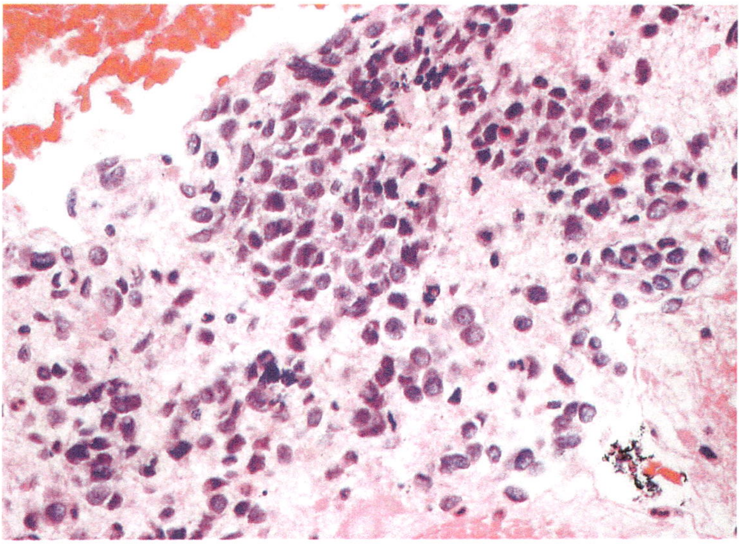

Fig. 8.13 Resected primary small cell carcinoma (SmCC) of the urinary bladder confirms the cytology described in Fig. 8.16. These tumors are characterized by small highly irregular nuclei 2–3 times the size of a lymphocyte nucleus. Tight nuclear groups frequently exhibit nuclei pushing into one another ("nuclear molding"). Histomorphology is similar to SmCC from other sites (*H&E, high mag.*)

Definition of SmCC

Malignant tumor of NE origin is similar to SmCC of lung and other sites. Tumor cells are positive for NE markers (synaptophysin, chromogranin, CD56) (Fig. 8.14).

Criteria

- Cellularity is usually moderate to high.
- Background is hemorrhagic and necrotic with single-cell necrosis (apoptosis), isolated or small groups of small, undifferentiated malignant cells, mitoses, and numerous polymorphonuclear leukocytes.
- Cells are arranged singly, in linear pattern, rosettes, loosely or tightly cohesive clusters (Fig. 8.15).
- Tumor cells are round to oval or irregular and small to medium in size (2–3 times the size of lymphocytes).
- Nuclei are small to oval, hyperchromatic with finely granular evenly distributed or smudged chromatin, ill-defined membranes, prominent molding, and display crush artifact. Nucleoli are absent or inconspicuous (Fig. 8.16).
- Cytoplasm is scanty
- N/C ratio is high.

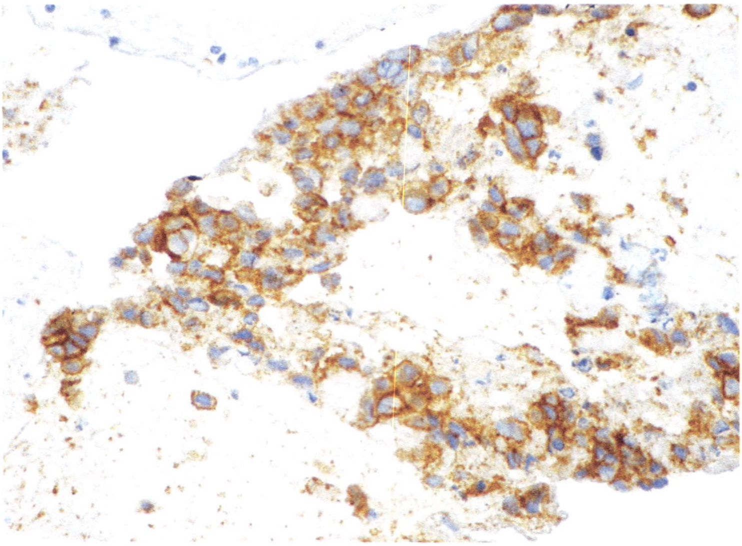

Fig. 8.14 Positive immunostain for CD56 (neural cell adhesion molecule, also found associated with skeletal muscle and NK cells) performed on the resected SmCC from the case described in Fig. 8.13 indicates the tumor's NE lineage (*Biopsy, IHC, high mag.*)

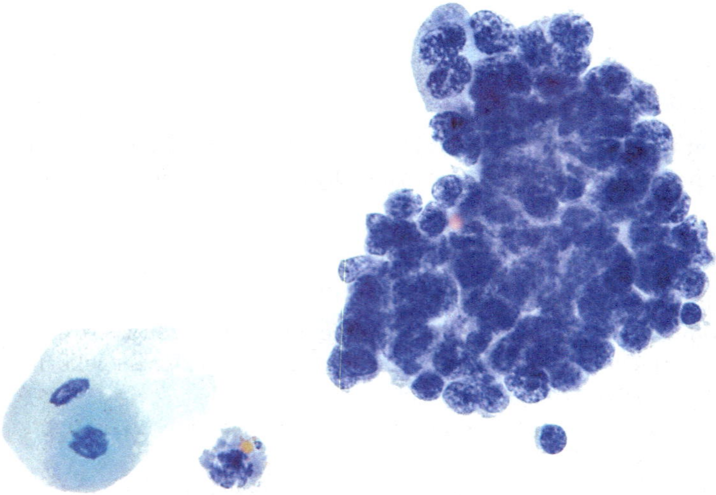

Fig. 8.15 A case of SmCC (histology depicted in Figs. 8.13 and 8.14) displays cells arranged in a tightly cohesive cluster. The background is clean and the typical crush artifact in these delicate cells is not evident. Tumor cells show a high nucleus-cytoplasmic ratio, moderately enlarged (compare to a lymphocyte at 5 o'clock position) round to oval irregular nuclei with hyperchromatic to smudged chromatin and absent or inconspicuous nucleoli. Nuclear overlap is more pronounced than molding. Cytoplasm is scant. Note benign umbrella cell in the *lower left corner* (*Voided urine, TP, high mag.*)

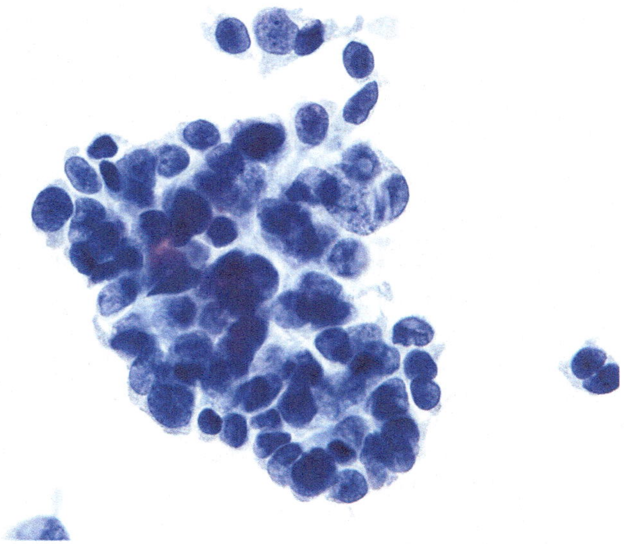

Fig. 8.16 Another case of SmCC displays cells arranged in a loosely-cohesive cluster. Other cytological features are similar to Fig. 8.15 (*Voided urine, TP, high mag.*)

LBPs [6, 18] (see Figs. 8.15 and 8.16)

- Cellularity is higher than conventional cytology
- Cleaner background with less inflammatory infiltrate. Granular necrotic debris appears clumped and clings to tumor cell clusters. Single malignant cells may be embedded in necrotic clumps.
- Preservation of above architectural features.
- Better preservation of cellular and nuclear details.
- Tumor cells are smaller than those seen in conventional preparations and rounder.
- Crush artifact may be less or represented by nuclear elongation.
- Nuclei show significant overlap, minimal or no molding and occasional micronucleoli.
- Cytoplasm is discernible, but scanty.

Explanatory Notes

Explanatory Note 1: Urine cytology has a low sensitivity and specificity for detecting SmCC, particularly, in cases intermixed with a UC cell component. The cytomorphology appears to be similar to SmCC of other sites [6, 18, 19].

Explanatory Note 2: An advantage of LBP, in addition to the better morphology, is the ability to perform immunocytochemistry for NE differentiation.

Explanatory Note 3: The cytological differential diagnosis includes metastatic SmCC from the lung, poorly differentiated small cell type SqCC, carcinoid, LCNEC, UC, lymphoma, melanoma, and other small cell malignancies. The NECs can be distinguished from carcinoid by the presence of tumor background and single-cell necrosis, frequent mitoses, and more nuclear atypia in SmCC and large high grade neoplastic cells in LCNEC. Thyroid transcription factor-1 (TTF-1) can be positive in 30 % of SmCC of the bladder and its positivity is still not certain in LCNEC. Other benign conditions such as inflammatory infiltrate, follicular cystitis, and BCG-associated changes should also be considered in the differential diagnosis [17]. Timely and accurate cytological diagnosis of SmCC is important to ensure a prompt clinical workup for these highly aggressive tumors. Mixed SmCC with conventional UC may be simply diagnosed as UC in urine cytology, if the SmCC cells are not sampled or masked by the conventional UC component.

Primary LCNEC of the urinary bladder is extremely rare with less than 20 reported cases in the surgical pathology literature [17]. Urinary cytological findings are similar to those described for LCNEC of the lung [20]. To make an unequivocal diagnosis of LCNEC, NE markers are mandated.

The cytological differential diagnosis and clinical behavior, management, and prognosis are similar to SmCC [19].

Non-Epithelial Malignancies

Sarcoma

Spindle cell lesions of the urinary bladder are uncommon and can pose a diagnostic challenge when encountered in urine cytology due to a vast differential diagnosis. These entities include benign processes such as pseudosarcomatous myofibroblastic proliferation encompassing lesions occurring either spontaneously or after instrumentation. Malignant tumors include sarcomatoid UC, leiomyosarcoma, angiosarcoma, and unclassified sarcoma. Sarcomas represent the most common mesenchymal tumors of the bladder and generally share an extremely aggressive biologic behavior, regardless of the histologic subtype. They clinically present with gross, painless hematuria. Presence of spindle cells in the urine indicate the need for a more invasive procedure to arrive at a correct diagnosis as a comprehensive panel of immunohistochemical stains may not be possible on a limited cytological sample. Moreover, surgical margin status at resection is an important determinant of survival [21].

Leiomyosarcoma. Leiomyosarcoma is the most common malignant mesenchymal tumor of the urinary bladder in adults, accounting for 1 % of all bladder malignancies [22]. Urine cytology shows sheets or scattered large atypical spindle cells with a moderate amount of ill-defined cytoplasm, large hyperchromatic and irregular nuclei with occasional nucleoli and a low nuclear cytoplasmic ratio (Fig. 8.17). Histological assessment (Fig. 8.18) and immunohistochemical positivity for smooth muscle actin (SMA) and desmin may confirm the diagnosis. To make a diagnosis of leiomyosarcoma in limited samples, sarcomatoid carcinoma should always be in the differential diagnosis.

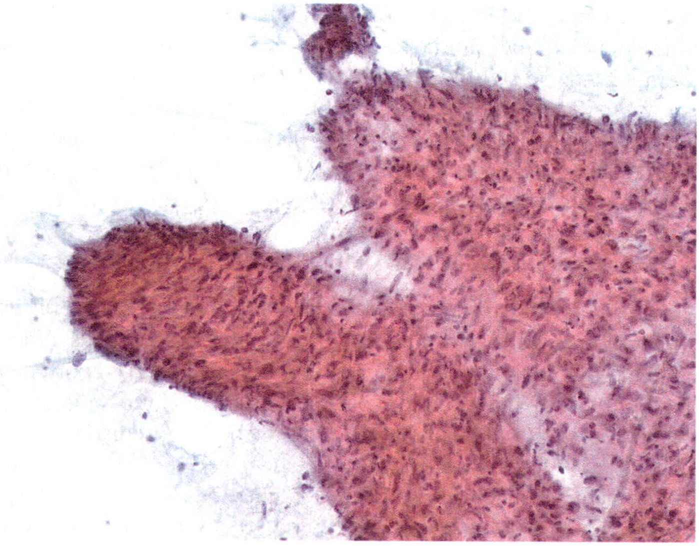

Fig. 8.17 Leiomyosarcoma of the urinary bladder shows fragments of atypical spindle cells amid stroma containing inflammatory cells. The cells contain large elongated ("cigar"-shaped) mildly hyperchromatic nuclei with a moderate amount of ill-defined cytoplasm (*Washing, CS, low mag.*)

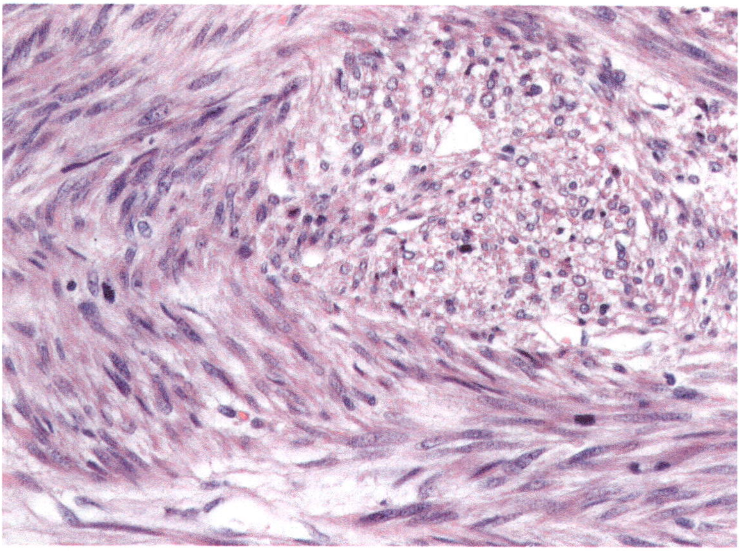

Fig. 8.18 Histology of the resected leiomyosarcoma from the above case demonstrates bundles of spindle-shaped cells in profile and cross-section with elongated and pleomorphic nuclei (*Biopsy, H&E, medium mag.*)

Sarcomatoid carcinoma is a relatively rare high grade neoplasm of the urinary bladder showing both malignant epithelial and mesenchymal differentiation. It is considered to be a variant of UC [23]. Computed tomography and magnetic resonance images show increased thickness of the bladder wall associated with a polypoid mass. The cytology of voided urine smears shows biphasic tumor cell populations with UC cells and spindle pleomorphic sarcomatoid malignant cells. On immunoperoxidase staining, the sarcomatoid cells show epithelial markers (cytokeratin [AE1/AE3], as well as mesenchymal markers vimentin, EMA, SMA, p53, S-100, CEA, and nuclear positivity for MIB1 [50 % labeled] positivity).

Angiosarcoma. Angiosarcomas are rare vascular neoplasms; visceral involvement is quite uncommon. Primary angiosarcoma of the bladder has not been well-characterized histologically due to its rarity with less than 20 reported cases in the English literature. Ionizing radiation, particularly therapeutic radiation and chemical agents such as vinyl chloride are thought to be the predisposing factors. The tumors tend to arise from all areas of the bladder and are aggressive with a short disease course. The most common clinical presentation is hematuria. Angiosarcoma of the bladder is more common in men with reports of male:female ratio of 8:1. As with most sarcomas, the lung and the liver are common sites for metastases, with a hematogenous metastatic pattern [24].

Cytological recognition may be difficult. The tumor cells can be spindled or epithelioid, arranged in nests and as single cells. The nuclei may be round to oval, large, irregular, hyperchromatic with prominent cherry-red nucleoli (Fig. 8.19). Cytoplasm is abundant, and may contain intracellular lumina containing erythrocytes. Mitosis and necrosis may be seen [24]. Histologic assessment and positive immunohistochemical staining for CD31, CD34, ERG, and Factor VIII is confirmatory (Figs. 8.20 and 8.21). Positive cytokeratin staining may lead to the false diagnosis of poorly differentiated carcinoma [24].

Hematologic Malignancy

Lymphoma (Fig. 8.22 and 8.23), plasmacytoma or multiple myeloma can be detected in urinary tract cytology [25, 26]. Since lymphoma-like or plasmacytoid UC has been well described, when one sees these morphologies, before rendering a diagnosis of lymphoma or plasmacytoma, UC variant should be excluded. Confirmatory flow cytometry and biopsy are usually essential for accurate characterization.

Melanoma

Primary melanoma of the bladder is very rare and secondary melanoma is more common. [27] Metastatic melanoma may present with melanuria and melanosis.

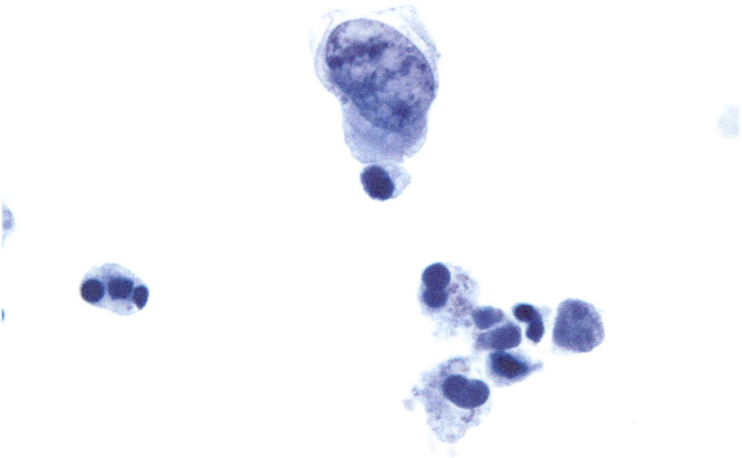

Fig. 8.19 Angiosarcoma of the urinary bladder displays a large anaplastic plump spindle cell in the upper mid-portion of the image, amid an inflammatory background. Other singly-dispersed and small groups of anaplastic malignant cells are also present. The large nucleus is oval and irregular with vesicular clumped chromatin and moderate amounts of pale cytoplasm. Confirmation of the diagnosis requires histological and immunochemical assessment. Malignancy is not a diagnostic issue (*Voided urine, TP, high mag.*)

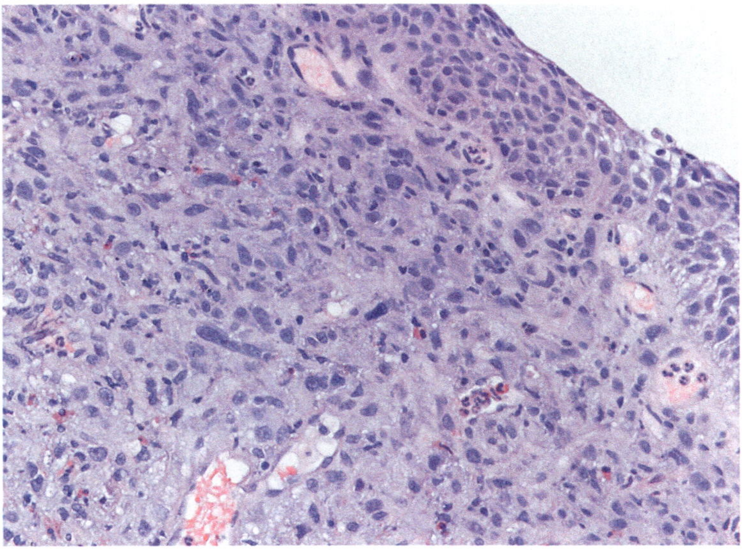

Fig. 8.20 Histology of the resected angiosarcoma of urinary bladder from the above case shows spindled and epithelioid cells arranged in nests and clusters interspersed with gaping small vascular channels lined by atypical endothelial cells. As is true of anaplastic sarcoma in other sites, angiosarcoma must be kept in the differential diagnosis. Surface urothelium is located at the upper right (*Biopsy, H&E, medium mag.*)

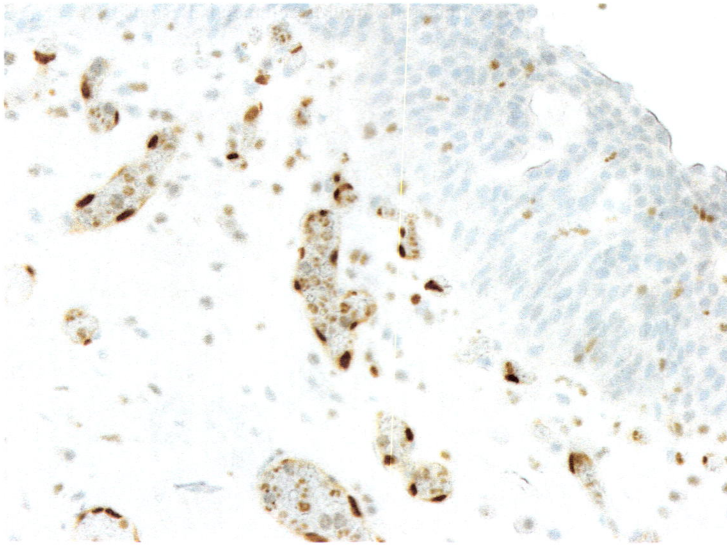

Fig. 8.21 Positive immunostaining for ERG (Erythroblast transformation specific Related Gene) confirms the above case as angiosarcoma (*Biopsy, IHC, medium mag.*)

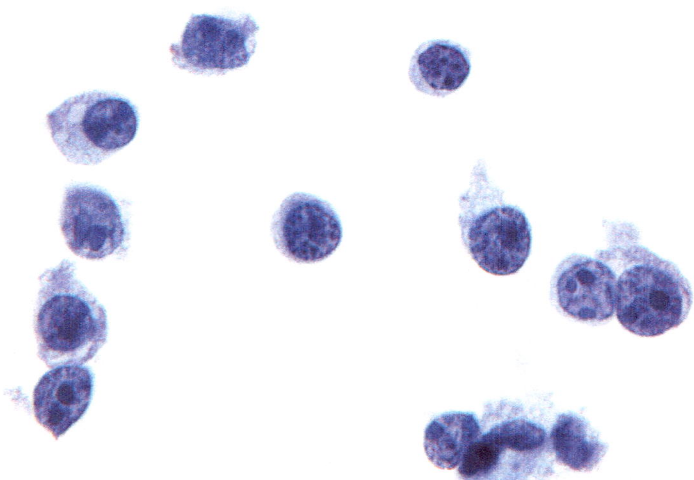

Fig. 8.22 Diffuse large B-cell lymphoma (DLBCL) involving the urinary bladder displays medium to large cells with round to oval nuclei, distinct smooth or irregular contours, vesicular chromatin and multiple prominent nucleoli, often peripheral. Cytoplasm is basophilic and vacuolated. Poorly differentiated carcinoma and conventional UC may mimic DLBCL (*Voided urine, TP, high mag.*)

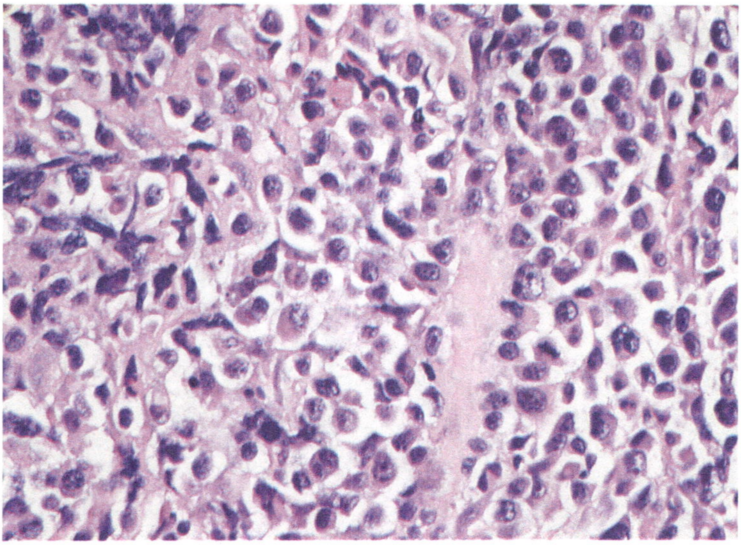

Fig. 8.23 Histology of the biopsied DLBCL from the above case, showing a cellular field of highly malignant crowded neoplastic cells. *(H&E, high mag.)*

Cytomorphologic findings of melanoma are individually scattered large atypical cells with round to oval nuclei with abundant cytoplasm. Nuclei are large, eccentric, and have prominent nucleoli with occasional nuclear pseudoinclusions. The cytoplasm may contain dark dusty brown melanin pigment (Fig. 8.24) [27].

Direct Extension and Metastatic Tumors to Urinary bladder

Background

Urinary bladder metastases from the solid tumors represent approximately 2 % of all bladder neoplasms. Involvement of the bladder by tumors from other organs occurs as either a metastasis or a direct extension [28]. Distant metastasis to the bladder is very rare, and is typically a late complication of the primary disease. Direct extension to the bladder from malignancies in adjacent organs, including colorectum, prostate, and female genital tract is much more frequent. The site of the tumor within the bladder may suggest its origin; for example, the cancers of the prostate and uterine cervix tend to invade the neck and trigone, while colorectal cancers more commonly involve the fundus [28].

Metastasis or direct extension of tumors can mimic UC or non-UC both cytologically and histologically. The rarity and overlap of cytomorphologic features make the cytological diagnosis difficult. The combination of accurate clinical information, cystoscopic findings, and ancillary tests including immunocytochemical staining enable confirmation of the diagnosis.

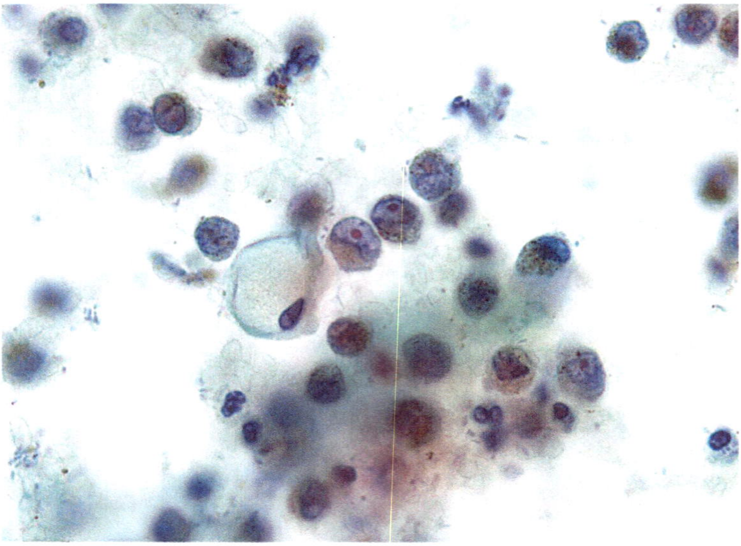

Fig. 8.24 Melanoma metastatic to urinary bladder shows individually scattered large atypical cells with round to oval nuclei with abundant cytoplasm. Nuclei are large, eccentric, and have prominent macronucleoli with occasional nuclear pseudoinclusions. The cytoplasm contains dark dusty brown melanin pigment (*Voided urine, TP, high mag.*)

Direct Extension (Carcinomas of Prostate, Colon, Rectum, Uterine Cervix)

AdCa of Prostate

Diagnostic value of prostatic AdCa in routine exfoliative cytology is limited because cytologically detected cases of prostatic AdCa are at a clinically advanced stage, and of a high Gleason score [29]. Hematuria and/or outlet obstruction are often presenting symptoms.

Cytologic features of conventional acinar prostatic AdCa show fragments of uniform, large cuboidal cells arranged in acinar formation with central lumens and azurophilic cytoplasm. The chromatin is typically fine with distinct nuclear membranes, and prominent nucleoli. Nuclei may be eccentrically placed. Background is usually clean.

Most helpful findings to differentiate prostatic AdCa from high grade UC are an oval to round nucleus with smooth borders, fine powdery, evenly distributed nuclear chromatin and a large prominent nucleolus when present, and lack of significant pleomorphism. However prostatic duct AdCa is difficult to differentiate from colorectal AdCa [29] or primary enteric type AdCa of the bladder. Ancillary immunocytochemistry for prostate-specific antigen, alpha-methylacyl-coA racemase (AMACR), and ERG immunostaining may be helpful for confirmative diagnosis [28, 29].

Colorectal AdCa

Cytologic findings of colorectal AdCa are elongated or columnar cells with pencil-shaped nuclei and gland formation, coarse chromatin, often inconspicuous nucleoli, and frequent tumor necrosis in background. The cells are pleomorphic, with degenerated hyperchromatic, irregular nuclear borders, and frequent cytoplasmic vacuolation. It is often indistinguishable from those of high grade UC and primary AdCa of the bladder. Immunohistochemical profile with CK20, beta-catenin, CDX-2, PSA, and PSAP may help in the diagnosis of colorectal origin [4, 30]. However, correlation with clinical history is mandatory.

SqCC of Uterine Cervix

SqCC from the uterine cervix is one of the common malignancies in lower female genital tract. Invasive SqCC of the cervix or of bladder origin may involve neighboring organs. Metastatic SqCC is difficult to differentiate from UC with squamous cell differentiation, and pure SqCC of the bladder. Clinical findings with ancillary test such as immunohistochemistry are necessary for differential diagnosis. P16 is diffusely expressed in most cervical SqCC, but diagnostic value is limited, because about 37 % of SqCC of urothelial origin also express p16 and UC is also positive for p16 [31]. Immunopositivity for CK14, desmoglein for SqCC and GATA3, uroplakin, S100P and thrombomodulin for UC is useful for differential diagnosis of SqCC from UC [31, 32].

Metastatic Tumors (Renal Cell, Breast, Ovarian, Lung, Stomach and Skin Carcinoma, Melanoma and Hematologic Malignancies)

Renal Cell Carcinoma (RCC)

Diagnostic value of RCC in urinary tract cytology is questionable because an actual metastasis to the bladder is very rare. Most of the reported bladder metastases of RCC are clear cell type; therefore, it is important to distinguish metastatic RCC from UC with clear cell features [4]. Cytomorphologic findings of RCC are tumor cells with vacuolar cytoplasm, granular chromatin, prominent nucleoli, and often clustered or gland-like arrangement. Multinucleated giant cells and cells with eccentric nuclei are also described. Granular eosinophilic cells with pyknotic nuclei and indistinct cytoplasmic borders are believed to be the results of degenerative changes caused by the urinary environment.

Breast Carcinoma

Metastatic breast carcinoma is frequently lobular type. Lobular carcinoma retains its cytological features and has tumor cells arranged in a linear (single file) configuration or small groups of cells. Individual cells are small with an eccentrically placed nucleus, small nucleolus, and vacuolated cytoplasm with occasional mucinous condensation ("targetoid" body) that recapitulate the histologic appearance (Figs. 8.25 and 8.26). Ductal carcinoma may also rarely be seen (Fig. 8.27). Clinical history with additional ancillary immunocytochemical stain for mammaglobin, GCDFP-15, GATA-3 may be helpful. GATA-3 shows diffuse moderate to strong nuclear staining in metastatic lobular carcinoma and may not be useful, if used alone, in distinguishing it from primary signet ring cell carcinoma of the bladder [33].

Gastric Carcinoma

Metastatic gastric cancer commonly shows signet ring cell morphology and requires differential diagnosis from a primary signet ring cell carcinoma of the bladder. Nuclear GATA-3 positivity is seen in primary AdCas of the urinary bladder with signet ring features and can be helpful in distinguishing it from gastric signet ring carcinomas [30].

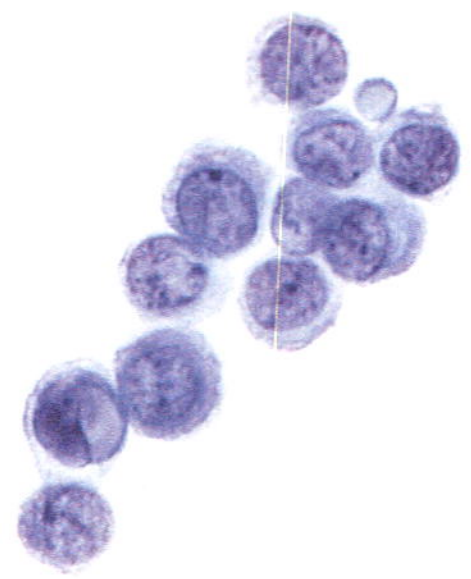

Fig. 8.25 Lobular breast carcinoma metastatic to urinary bladder shows tumor cells arranged in a small group with focal linear ("Indian file") configuration. Individual cells are small with an eccentrically placed nucleus, small nucleolus, and occasionally vacuolated cytoplasm (*Voided urine, TP, high mag.*)

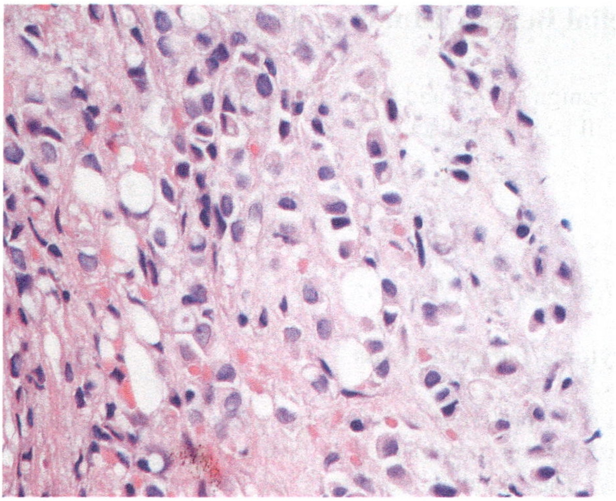

Fig. 8.26 Histology of the biopsied lobular carcinoma of breast from the above case demonstrates neoplastic cells from lobular percolating through the connective tissue, often in linear array (*H&E, high mag.*)

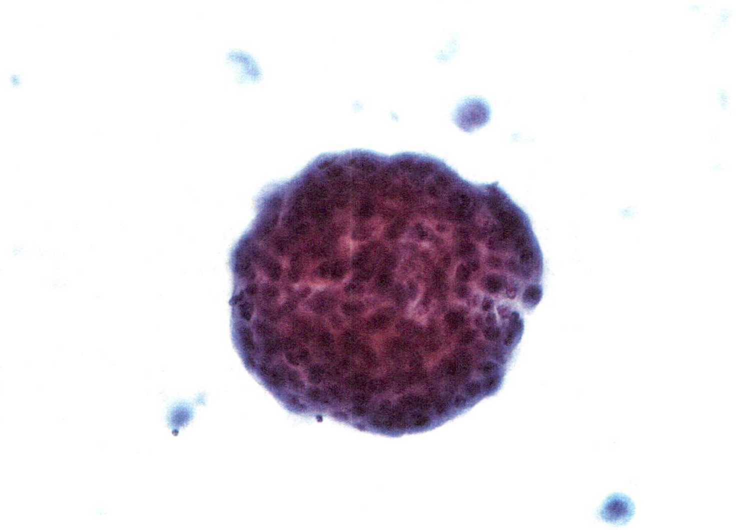

Fig. 8.27 Metastatic ductal carcinoma of the breast shows tumor cells forming a cellular sphere ("morula") that is typical of these tumors in liquid specimens (*Voided urine, TP, high mag.*)

Non-Epithelial Benign Tumors and Tumor-Like Conditions

Non-epithelial benign tumors and tumor-like conditions are extremely rare and only a few lesions will be briefly discussed [14]. Readers are referred to specialty books for details.

Non-Epithelial Benign Tumors

Pheochromocytoma/Paraganglioma

Paraganglioma is the preferred term for extra-adrenal pheochromocytoma. Primary paragangliomas of the urinary bladder are rare and comprise less than 0.05 % of all bladder tumors. They tend to be functional and occur mostly in young adult Caucasians. The most common symptoms and signs of paraganglioma of the urinary bladder are hypertension, headache, and hematuria. They are usually treated by partial cystectomy. Patients with localized tumors are treated with less aggressive modalities and have a favorable prognosis, while patients with metastatic disease have a significant reduction in survival rates despite aggressive treatment [34].

Tumor-Like Lesions

Nephrogenic Adenoma

Nephrogenic adenoma is an uncommon, benign, tumor-like lesion within the urothelial mucosa most commonly of the urinary bladder. It is considered to be of renal tubular cell origin and associated with chronic irritation of the mucosa, by injury, infection, calculi, post-instrumentation, or renal transplantation. Middle-aged men are more commonly affected; gross hematuria, dysuria, and frequency are the usual presenting symptoms. Urinary cytology may show cuboidal to low columnar cells with scant cytoplasm, but cells with abundant clear cytoplasm may also be seen. Nuclear atypia is not evident. Histologically, tubular, cystic, and polypoid to papillary patterns are the most common characteristics lined by a single layer of cells as described above. Haphazard distribution of tubules and clear cytoplasm may simulate adenocarcinoma such as prostate or RCC. Diagnostic difficulties may be resolved by immunohistochemistry [14].

Amyloidosis

Primary localized amyloidosis of the urinary bladder is a rare disease that clinically, radiologically, and cystoscopically mimics primary bladder malignancy. Patients usually present with intermittent gross hematuria. Urine cytology may show clumps of amorphous material. Confirmation of amyloidosis usually requires bladder biopsy. Treatment includes fulguration or laser for small localized lesions and transurethral resection or partial cystectomy for larger lesions [35].

Inflammatory Pseudotumor (Pseudosarcomatous Fibromyxoid Tumor)

These lesions are also referred to as inflammatory myofibroblastic tumor postoperative spindle cell nodule of the bladder, and are unusual lesions of uncertain pathogenesis that share overlapping, if not identical, histologic features. Inflammatory pseudotumor (pseudosarcomatous fibromyxoid tumor; inflammatory myofibroblastic tumor) is usually considered to be of reactive or occur post-instrumentation or surgery. The mean age is 47 years with a male predominance. Hematuria is the common presentation. Grossly the lesions present as polypoid or nodular masses and involve any portion of the bladder wall, with a mean size of 4 cm. Histologically they are composed of spindled and stellate cells arranged in a myxoid background with numerous inflammatory cells. Cytologically, bland spindle cells with elongated nuclei and prominent nucleoli may be seen [14].

References

1. Dahm P, Gschwend JE. Malignant non-urothelial neoplasms of the urinary bladder: a review. Eur Urol. 2003;44:672–81. Review.
2. Chalasani V, Chin JL, Izawa JI. Histologic variants of urothelial bladder cancer and nonurothelial histology in bladder cancer. Can Urol Assoc J. 2009;3(6 Suppl 4):S193–8.
3. Abol-Enein H, Kava BR, Carmack AJ. Nonurothelial cancer of the bladder. Urology. 2007;69 (1 Suppl):93–104. Review.
4. Xiao GQ, Chow J, Unger PD. Metastatic tumors to the urinary bladder: clinicopathologic study of 11 cases. Int J Surg Pathol. 2012;20:342–8.
5. Laucirica R, Bentz JS, Souers RJ, Wasserman PG, Crothers BA, Clayton AC, et al. Do liquid-based preparations of urinary cytology perform differently than classically prepared cases? Observations from the College of American Pathologists Interlaboratory Comparison Program in Nongynecologic Cytology. Arch Pathol Lab Med. 2010;134:19–22.
6. Hoda RS. Non-gynecologic cytology on liquid-based preparations: a morphologic review of facts and artifacts. Diagn Cytopathol. 2007;35:621–34. Review.
7. Koss LG, Hoda RS. Koss's cytology of the urinary tract with histopathologic correlations. New York: Springer Press; 2012.
8. Khaled H. Schistosomiasis and cancer in Egypt: review. J Adv Res. 2013;4:461–6.
9. Hattori M, Nishimura Y, Toyonaga M, Kakinuma H, Matsumoto K, Ohbu M. Cytological significance of abnormal squamous cells in urinary cytology. Diagn Cytopathol. 2012;40:798–803.
10. Gulmann C, Paner GP, Parakh RS, Hansel DE, Shen SS, Ro JY, et al. Immunohistochemical profile to distinguish urothelial from squamous differentiation in carcinomas of urothelial tract. Hum Pathol. 2013;44:164–72.
11. Zhong M, Gersbach E, Rohan SM, Yang XJ. Primary adenocarcinoma of the urinary bladder: differential diagnosis and clinical relevance. Arch Pathol Lab Med. 2013;137:371–81.
12. Bardales RH, Pitman MB, Stanley MW, Korourian S, Suhrland MJ. Urine cytology of primary and secondary urinary bladder adenocarcinoma. Cancer. 1998;84:335–43.
13. Guan H, Tatsas AD, Ali SZ. Signet ring cell carcinoma in urine cytology: cytomorphologic findings and differential diagnosis. Acta Cytol. 2012;56:177–82.

14. Young RH. Tumor-like lesions of the urinary bladder. Mod Pathol. 2009;22 Suppl 2:S37–52.
15. Ellis CL, Chang AG, Cimino-Mathews A, Argani P, Youssef RF, Kapur P, et al. GATA-3 immunohistochemistry in the differential diagnosis of adenocarcinoma of the urinary bladder. Am J Surg Pathol. 2013;37:1756–60.
16. Chen YB, Epstein JI. Primary carcinoid tumors of the urinary bladder and prostatic urethra: a clinicopathologic study of 6 cases. Am J Surg Pathol. 2011;35:442–6.
17. Alijo Serrano F, Sánchez-Mora N, Angel Arranz J, Hernández C, Alvarez-Fernández E. Large cell and small cell neuroendocrine bladder carcinoma: immunohistochemical and outcome study in a single institution. Am J Clin Pathol. 2007;128:733–9.
18. Ciesla MC, Guidos BJ, Selvaggi SM. Cytomorphology of small-cell (neuroendocrine) carcinoma on ThinPrep cytology as compared to conventional smears. Diagn Cytopathol. 2001;24:46–52.
19. Helpap B. Morphology and therapeutic strategies for neuroendocrine tumors of the genitourinary tract. Cancer. 2002;95:1415–20.
20. Acs G, Gupta PK, Baloch ZW. Cytomorphology of high-grade neuroendocrine carcinoma of the urinary tract. Diagn Cytopathol. 2000;23:92–6.
21. Westfall DE, Folpe AL, Paner GP, Oliva E, Goldstein L, Alsabeh R, et al. Utility of a comprehensive immunohistochemical panel in the differential diagnosis of spindle cell lesions of the urinary bladder. Am J Surg Pathol. 2009;33:99–105.
22. Hemachandran M, Nada R, Rajwanshi A. Leiomyosarcoma of the urinary bladder: a diagnostic challenge in urine cytology. Diagn Cytopathol. 2004;31:281–2.
23. Iwa N, Ito S, Takegaki Y, Ikura Y, Kobayashi TK, Yasukawa S, Kobayashi Y. Cytologic features of sarcomatoid carcinoma of the urinary bladder: a case report. Diagn Cytopathol. 2013;41:536–41.
24. Schindler S, De Frias DV, Yu GH. Primary angiosarcoma of the bladder: cytomorphology and differential diagnosis. Cytopathology. 1999;10:137–43.
25. Cheson BD, Schumann JL, Schumann GB. Urinary cytodiagnostic abnormalities in 50 patients with non-Hodgkin's lymphomas. Cancer. 1984;54:1914–9.
26. Jiménez-Hernández M, López-Guillermo A, Cobo F, Bladé J, Aguilar JL, Villamor N, Montserrat E. Bladder involvement of diffuse large B-cell lymphoma diagnosed by a cytological study of the urine. Leuk Lymphoma. 2002;43:187–9.
27. Khalbuss WE, Hossain M, Elhosseiny A. Primary malignant melanoma of the urinary bladder diagnosed by urine cytology: a case report. Acta Cytol. 2001;45:631–5.
28. Velcheti V, Govindan R. Metastatic cancer involving bladder: a review. Can J Urol. 2007;14:3443–8. Review.
29. Sathiyamoorthy S, Ali SZ. Urinary cytology of prostatic duct adenocarcinoma: a clinicopathologic analysis. Acta Cytol. 2013;57:184–8.
30. Rao Q, Williamson SR, Lopez-Beltran A, Montironi R, Huang W, Eble JN, et al. Distinguishing primary adenocarcinoma of the urinary bladder from secondary involvement by colorectal adenocarcinoma: extended immunohistochemical profiles emphasizing novel markers. Mod Pathol. 2013;26:725–32.
31. Blochin EB, Park KJ, Tickoo SK, Reuter VE, Al-Ahmadie H. Urothelial carcinoma with prominent squamous differentiation in the setting of neurogenic bladder: role of human papillomavirus infection. Mod Pathol. 2012;25:1534–42.
32. Gailey MP, Bellizzi AM. Immunohistochemistry for the novel markers glypican 3, PAX8, and p40 (DeltaNp63) in squamous cell and urothelial carcinoma. Am J Clin Pathol. 2013;140:872–80.
33. Liu H, Shi J, Wilkerson ML, Lin F. Immunohistochemical evaluation of GATA3 expression in tumors and normal tissues: a useful immunomarker for breast and urothelial carcinomas. Am J Clin Pathol. 2012;138:57–64.
34. Beilan JA, Lawton A, Hajdenberg J, Rosser CJ. Pheochromocytoma of the urinary bladder: a systematic review of the contemporary literature. BMC Urol. 2013;13:22–8.
35. Akram CM, Al-Marhoon MS, Mathew J, Grant CS, Rao TV. Primary localized AA type amyloidosis of urinary bladder: case report of rare cause of episodic painless hematuria. Urology. 2006;68:1343. e15-7.

Chapter 9
Ancillary Studies in Urinary Cytology

Lukas Bubendorf, Nancy P. Caraway, Andrew H. Fischer, Ruth L. Katz, Matthew T. Olson, Fernando Schmitt, Margareta Strojan Fležar, Theodorus H. Van Der Kwast, and Philippe Vielh

Background

The difficulties and challenges of urinary cytology have been driving the search for biomarkers and development of commercial diagnostic assays to improve its sensitivity for detecting urothelial carcinoma (UC). Over the last two decades, the number of review articles on urinary markers for detection of bladder cancer has steeply risen. Despite the countless markers that have been proposed, only a few have reached the stage of approved assays for diagnostic application. Evaluation of individual markers has been hindered by the complexity of the disease diagnosis and behavior, the various clinical endpoints, and the different types of treatment dependent upon tumor grade and stage. Importantly, many studies have been done without reference to matched cytology results. Interpretation of published studies is difficult because cytological findings and results of ancillary tests often cannot be linked back to particular stages and grades of UC. These factors make it at least challenging if not impossible to define an optimal role for ancillary studies through review of the literature. Concerns about cost-effectiveness of ancillary testing are another source of ongoing discussions. For these reasons, no single ancillary test is clearly being recommended as part of the routine evaluation in the Guidelines of the American Urological Association and the European Association of Urology at this time.

There are basically two types of ancillary tests: those that are based on cytological preparations (cell-based tests) and those that rely on a nonmorphologic analysis of urinary fluids (liquid-based tests). Both types of tests are reviewed in separate sections of this chapter. Liquid-based tests, such as NMP22, are mainly meant to be applied in the office of the urologists to identify patients with high risk of primary UC or recurrence, while the cytology-based tests are usually in the hands of cytology laboratories. Many of the controversies on the value of ancillary testing in urinary cytology are caused by the lack of clear indications.

D.L. Rosenthal et al. (eds.), *The Paris System for Reporting Urinary Cytology*, DOI 10.1007/978-3-319-22864-8_9

The Paris System for Reporting Urinary Cytology (The Paris System) provides an opportunity to define and narrow down the diagnostic categories in which ancillary testing of urinary specimens is most rewarding, and to avoid unnecessary testing in areas with minimal or no added value. The Paris System lays the ground for prospective studies in search of cost-effective combinations of urine cytologywith ancillary testing to improve diagnosis and clinical outcome of UC. While we will summarize several proposed diagnostic markers, we will place a special emphasis on two cell-based tests that have been approved by the U.S. Food and Drug Administration (FDA), UroVysion® (U-FISH; Abbott Laboratories, Abbott Park, IL, USA) and ImmunoCyt/UCyt+® (uCyt; Diagnocure Inc, Quebec, Canada). They are indicated for the diagnosis of UC in patients with hematuria and/or monitoring for tumor recurrence in patients previously diagnosed with bladder cancer. To date, U-FISH is considered the most promising ancillary test in urinary cytology and is therefore discussed in a separate section of this chapter [1]. This test is based on the detection of numerical and structural chromosomal aberrations, which are a hallmark of cancer but only rarely seen in benign cells. In contrast, the immunofluorescence-based test uCyt relies on the detection of three proteins that are preferentially expressed by UC cells as opposed to benign cells.

Pre-analytical Procedures, Technique, and Evaluation of UroVysion® FISH

The commercially available multitarget multicolor U-FISH assay contains four single-stranded DNA probes. Three probes are chromosome enumeration probes (CEP) targeting pericentromeric regions of chromosomes 3, 7, and 17. Another probe is a locus-specific identifier (LSI) probe targeting 9p21 locus on gene p16. All probes are directly labelled with fluorescent dyes, specifically CEP 3 SpectrumRed, CEP 7 SpectrumGreen, CEP 17 Spectrum Aqua, and LSI 9p21 SpectrumGold.

Specimen Preparation

The U-FISH test was originally intended for use on voided urine specimens. However, later studies have proved its use on other fluid specimens from the urinary tract, e.g., bladder washings and upper urinary tract (UUT) washings. Specimens from the urinary tract should be processed to fix cell preparations on glass slides as soon as possible after collection (within 3 h). If a delay in processing is anticipated, samples can be prefixed with 2 % polyethylene glycol in 50 % ethanol (Carbowax) or other preservatives (e.g., an equal volume of 50 % ethanol) and preferably processed within 72 h. Different techniques of slide preparation can be used for U-FISH test. The technique using 12-well slides, as suggested by the test manufacturer, is rarely used in the cytology laboratory. Common slide preparations include Cytospins in which a suspension of cells are centrifuged onto glass slides in a uniform monolayer 6 mm in diameter using a high speed centrifuge (Shandon Cytospin® 4 centrifuge, Thermo Fisher Scientific; Waltham, MA, USA). Smears of cell buttons after centrifugation, imprints of membrane filtration such as ThinPrep® (Hologic, Boxborough, MA), sedimentation of pre-processed urinary samples by SurePath® (Becton, Dickinson and Company, Franklin Lakes, NJ) are all acceptable. There should be 100–200 well-preserved cells in the target area for hybridization, and spread in monolayer. Slide preparations should be either air-dried or fixed by alcohol-based fixatives.

Unstained slide preparations are often used for the assay. However U-FISH is also applicable to slides that have originally been stained according to the Papanicolaou method to enable cytomorphological evaluation before the FISH assay. The area of interest with abnormal urothelial cells should be chosen and re-located for subsequent target hybridization, as described in more detail in the section on automation.

The basic principles of the U-FISH assay are illustrated in Fig. 9.1. In addition, The technical procedures including slide pretreatment and hybridization are described in the Appendix.

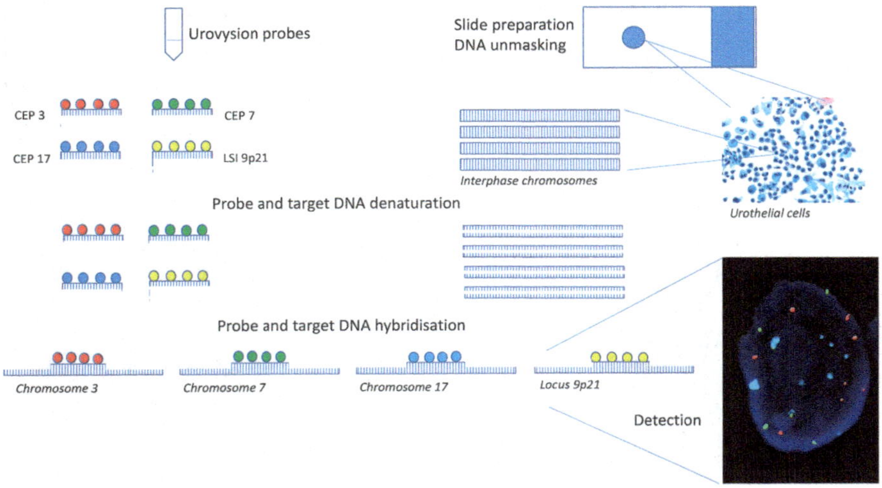

Fig. 9.1 Basic principles of U-FISH assay. The assay contains directly fluorescent dye-labelled single-strand DNA probes. Pre-analytical procedures include slide preparation (including pretreatment of pre-stained slides). UroVysion assay starts with probe preparation and specimen—target—DNA denaturation followed by DNA hybridization of probes to target DNA sequences. Analysis of FISH signals is performed under epifluorescent microscope. Legend: *CEP* centromere enumeration probe, *LSI* locus-specific identifier probe, *chr.* chromosome, *loc.* locus

Analysis of FISH Signals

An epi-fluorescence microscope equipped with a 100-watt mercury lamp and appropriate filters is recommended to detect multicolor fluorescent signals. Specimens should be scanned at 400× magnification to locate cells with nuclear signals and then analyzed under 600–1000× magnification. Systematic analysis of signals follows and a standardized and repeatable approach is essential (e.g., starting analysis in the upper left quadrant of the target area and continue scanning from left to right and top to bottom). Signals should be counted in abnormal cells, which are defined by their nuclear features, namely enlarged nuclear size, irregular nuclear borders, and "patchy" 4,6-diamidino, 2-phenylindole dihydrochloride (DAPI) staining. Besides the single cells, cell clusters may be evaluated avoiding counting signals in overlapping nuclei. The number of signals for all four probes should be counted for each abnormal cell and recorded only when there is a gain (≥2 signals) for two or more chromosomes 3 (red), 7 (green), 17 (aqua), or there is a loss of both copies of 9p21 (gold) as recommended by the manufacturer. Total number of abnormal cells analyzed should be recorded. The test is considered positive when ≥4 of the 25 analyzed cells show gains for two or more chromosomes or ≥12 of the 25 cells have zero 9p21 signals. If these criteria for test positivity are not met after viewing 25 cells, analysis should be continued until the entire sample is analyzed. Some authors have recommended optimization of the criteria with regard to the presence of benign tetraploid cells [2, 3]. Tetraploid, or less commonly octaploid, cells showing four or eight signals for each of the four FISH probes can occur in reactive cells (e.g., umbrella cells) and may give rise to false-positive FISH results. Thus, FISH results should not be considered positive based on a tetraploid pattern unless they are numerous (e.g., ≥10). Along this line, the FDA-approved package insert emphasizes that results at or near the cut-off point should be interpreted with caution. A schematic illustration of typical U-FISH findings is shown in Fig. 9.2.

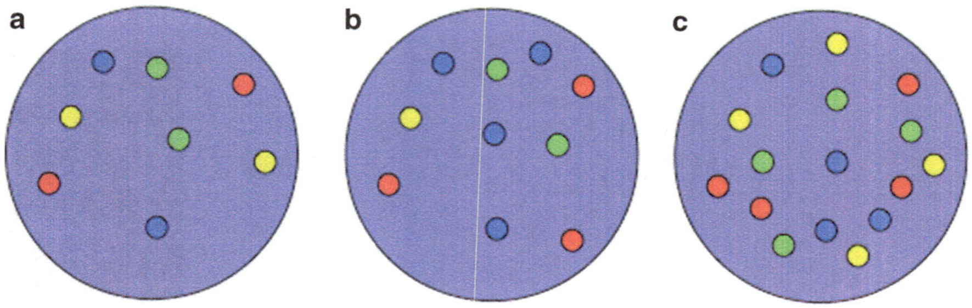

Fig. 9.2 Schematic illustration of U-FISH findings. (**a**) Nuclei of a FISH-negative benign cell with two signals for the chromosomes 3 (*red*), 7 (*green*), and 17 (*aqua*), and for 9p21 (*gold*). (**b**) U-FISH-positive cell with increased and unbalanced number of chromosomes 3 (*red*) and 17 (*aqua*) and heterozygous loss of 9p21 (*gold*). (**c**) Tetraploid FISH pattern with four signals of each FISH probe. This pattern is not specific for urothelial carcinoma but commonly seen in reactive urothelial cells

There are several conditions that may prevent accurate FISH examination, including the presence of lubricant jelly, corpora amylacea, degenerated cells, crystals, sperm, and bacteria.

In the case of performing FISH on conduit urines, interference by inflammation and cell debris may occur. Squamous contamination, especially in urines from female subjects, may obscure urothelial cells. If there are only a few atypical cells present, then a targeted FISH approach, using the same Papanicolaou-stained preparation as the cytology slide, is advisable.

Imaging and Automation of UroVysion® FISH Analysis

Advantages of an Automated Imaging System

Because manual FISH analysis has a relatively slow throughput and the fluorescent signals fade over time [4], automated imaging systems are increasingly being utilized, especially in institutions with high volumes of FISH tests. Reviewing representative digitized images instead of manual review of a FISH slide at a microscope can lead to dramatic savings in pathologist time [5]. Imaging systems may also be implemented for improved productivity, quality control, archiving of images, and increased accuracy. In a recent (2013) College of American Pathologists (CAP) proficiency test survey involving 192 laboratories, use of automated systems was estimated to be almost 50 %, with manual counting making up the remainder. In some labs there was a combination of both manual and automated use. In non-US countries, automated imaging systems for U-FISH analysis are less commonly used.

A high concordance (>98 %) between the manual method and the automated method of reviewing cells has been shown. In several cases deemed negative by the manual method, machine-assisted interpretation showed a positive result for abnormal cells which was subsequently verified within a short interval by cystoscopy [5]. In addition, the ability to enlarge cells with questionable signals and enhance weak signals is advantageous in reducing false-positive or false-negative results.

Disadvantages of automation may include a higher number of unsatisfactory specimens due to scant cellularity or clumping, in which case the manual system of review is employed. Factors to consider before purchasing an imaging system include financial cost, space requirements, information technology system needs or modifications, validation of system, training programs for personnel, continuing education, maintenance of system, workflow, and patterns of reimbursement [5].

Details of Automated Imaging Systems

Imaging systems consist of an automated scanning microscope coupled with software for image analysis. Some are approved or validated by the FDA for the detection, classification, and enumeration of urine specimen cells from individuals

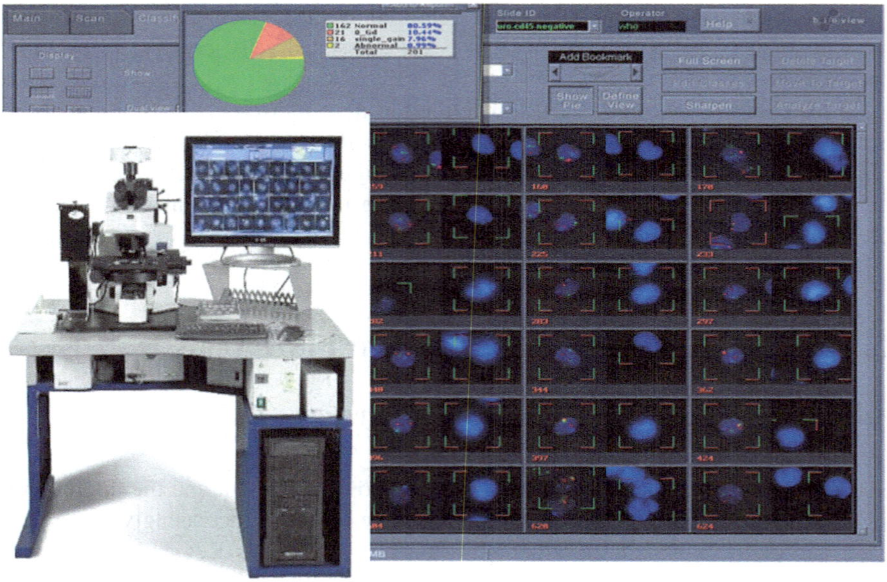

Fig. 9.3 Automated scanning instrument showing workstation with concurrent acquisition of DAPI images and FISH images illustrated on screen

with a history of UC probed by the U-FISH Kit. Imaging Systems that have been approved by the FDA (as of 2014). These include the Duet TM System™ (Bio View, LTD; Figs. 9.3 and 9.4) and the Ikoniscope oncoFISH Bladder Test System (Ikonsys, Inc., New Haven, Connecticut). Technical details of these imaging systems are described in the Appendix. Automated systems allow for interactive rejection or acceptance of cells, so that overlapping cells or degenerated cells can be ignored [6]. The imaged cells are then formatted in a gallery on a screen for review. Normal and abnormal cells can be segregated and then reclassified as needed [5]. Extraneous cells such as neutrophils and lymphocytes are automatically excluded from analysis.

Target FISH

FISH may also be performed on Papanicolaou-stained cytospins that have been pre-scanned by the imaging system with atypical urothelial cells selected by the operator. The slide is subsequently destained with acid alcohol and hybridized with the four-color probe set. The hybridized cells are then matched in perfect relocation with the pre-selected cells so that these same cells can be analyzed for abnormal

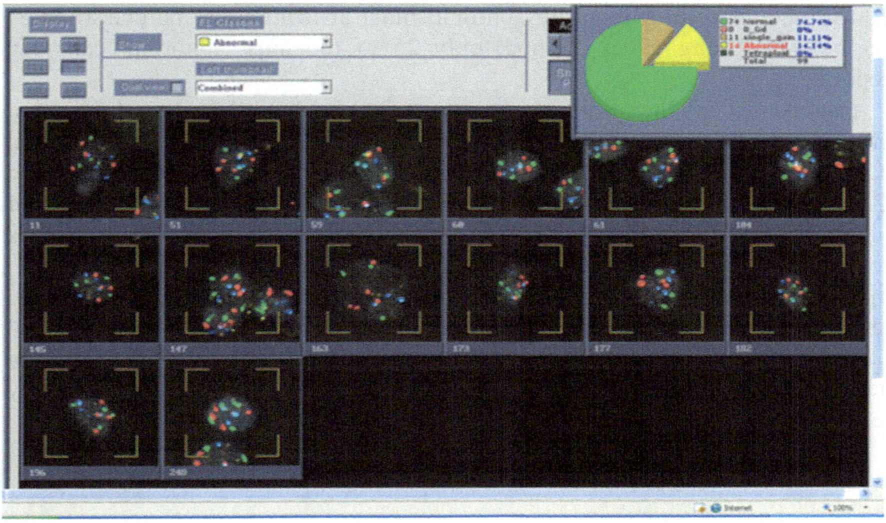

Fig. 9.4 Urine from a patient with a history of high grade urothelial carcinoma. Histogram of Urovysion FISH abnormal cells showing 14 out of 25 cells with polysomy for at least two chromosomes per cell. This is an abnormal result and consistent with high grade urothelial carcinoma. Although a total of 99 cells were scored, reporting is based on 25 of the most morphologically abnormal cells scored

FISH signals. This is also known as target FISH, and was shown to be more accurate when compared to conventional cytology [7]. In laboratories that do not have an automated imaging system in place, targeted U-FISH analysis of atypical urothelial cells can also be achieved by usage of a standard fluorescence microscope equipped with an automated stage and a camera allowing for interactive automated relocation and imaging of representative cells for review and documentation [8]. Target FISH enables the reviewer to associate aneuploidy with cytologic features on a per cell basis.

Reporting of Results

Following examination of all cells a report summarizing the sample's data is generated.

One or several pathologists can sign-out cases by using remote computers situated away from the main automated scanning microscope equipped with appropriate software [5, 9]. In manual screening a minimum of 25 abnormal cells are evaluated. In contrast, the automated systems require a minimum of

100 urothelial cells without any chromosomal aberrations to be classified as normal [5]. Using either method, only 25 of the most abnormal cells are reported.

Factors affecting the scanning performance include the cellularity, hybridization efficiency, and cleanliness of the slide and coverslip. In addition, slides with marked bacterial contamination [4] or obscuring inflammation are difficult to analyze. The CAP requires photographic or digitized images for all FISH assays which should include at least one cell image for assays with normal results and two cells images for assays with abnormal results (images of at least two cells are required to document all abnormalities since the multiple chromosome loci are evaluated in a single test). Images on all FISH assays testing for neoplastic conditions must be retained for documentation for a minimum of 10 years (CAP requirement CyG.43300). In addition, CAP requires that pathologists and technologists participate in proficiency testing [5].

Performance of UroVysion® FISH Testing

U-FISH testing of voided urine has been approved by the FDA as an aid for initial diagnosis of bladder cancer in patients with hematuria and/or subsequent monitoring for tumor recurrence in patients previously diagnosed with bladder cancer. In routine practice, there are several additional situations in which U-FISH is frequently used [8]. In a meta-analysis, the pooled sensitivity and specificity of FISH were 72 % and 83 %, respectively, as compared with 42 % and 96 %, respectively for cytology [10]. Putting published data of U-FISH results into the right perspective is challenging due to great variability of critical parameters; these include the type of specimen (voided urine versus bladder washing), clinical situation (history or no history of bladder cancer), concurrent cystoscopy findings, length and type of follow-up, proportion of low grade and high grade tumors, local experience in FISH analysis, and the definition of a positive result, among others. This emphasizes the need for a well-controlled and independently funded study to clarify the performance of FISH in clearly defined situations.

UroVysion FISH in Atypical Urinary Cytology

Atypical urinary cytology (AUC) has emerged as the most rewarding application of U-FISH analysis [2, 11–17]. In particular U-FISH is currently regarded as the most useful marker in the setting of a negative cystoscopy and atypical cytology according to the recent recommendations of the International Consultations on Urological Diseases and the European Society of Urology [1]. In a pivotal study,

U-FISH in 120 urine specimens revealed a sensitivity of 100, 89, and 60 % in patients with suspicious, atypical, and negative cytology, respectively, while the overall specificity was 97 % [18]. This is in line with another study showing that the sensitivity of FISH to detect UC in patients with atypical cytology and equivocal or negative cystoscopy was 100 % with a specificity ranging from 60 to 100 % depending on whether or not there was a history of UC or a lesion at cystoscopy [15]. The low positive predictive value in patients with a history of UC and a negative cystoscopy in this study were explained by early detection of neoplastic cells that preceded the appearance of established cancer. In fact, in other studies, such "anticipatory positive" FISH results predicted recurrence in patients under surveillance with atypical or suspicious cytology and a negative cystoscopy [16, 17, 19]. Despite these promising data, performing FISH after an AUC result and a negative surveillance cystoscopy is not yet generally recommended since these results are unlikely to change the currently established surveillance strategies in non-muscle-invasive UC.

U-FISH is particularly helpful in the notoriously difficult field of atypical cytology after intravesical BCG treatment of high grade non-muscle-invasive UC [12, 20–22]. Patients with a positive post-BCG cytology or FISH result have a substantially higher risk of recurrence when compared to patients with negative results [12, 23]. Washing cytologies of the UUT can also be challenging due to instrumentation-related changes that might lead to false-positive cytology results. On the other hand, accurate diagnosis of UUT UC is critical to avoid delay of diagnosis. Published reports suggest that U-FISH also appears as an interesting tool to increase the sensitivity for the detection of UC of the UUT (reviewed in [8]). In our experience, FISH is very helpful in atypical UUT washing cytology. However, one needs to be familiar with tetraploid U-FISH patterns that may occur in reactive conditions in order to avoid false-positive FISH diagnoses, as discussed below. Examples of U-FISH in atypical urinary cytology are shown in Fig. 9.5.

Cost-Effectiveness of UroVysion FISH

There have been concerns about the cost-effectiveness of the relatively expensive U-FISH testing, mainly because of the low positive predictive value. If applied to unselected patients with hematuria and recognizing the limited clinical value of enhanced detection of low grade UC, FISH results cost the patient a high price [8]. However, recent data suggest cost-effectiveness of negative U-FISH results following AUC results with equivocal or negative cystoscopy by avoiding unnecessary biopsies [13].

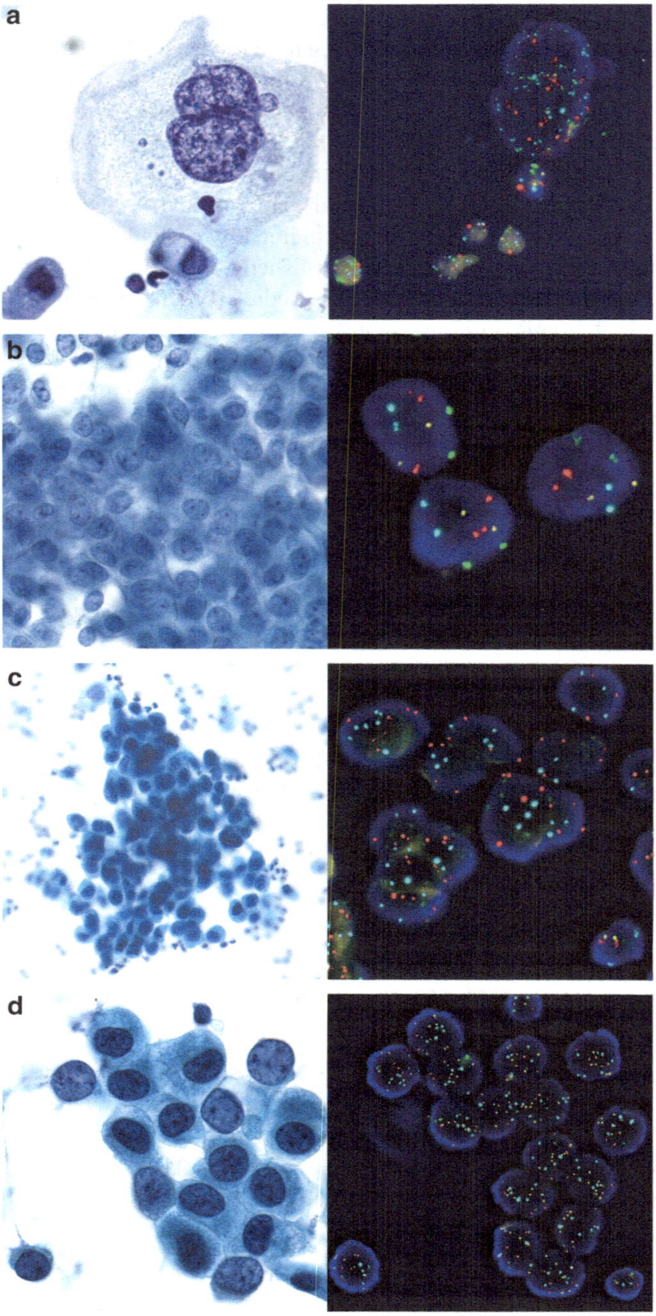

Fig. 9.5 Examples of UroVysion FISH and corresponding cytology (Papanicolaou stain) in urinary cytology. Chromosomes 3 in *red*, 7 in *green*, 17 in *aqua* and 9p21 in *gold*. (**a**) Benign bi- or multinucleate umbrella cell with pronounced reactive changes in a patient with irritative

Pitfalls in UroVysion® FISH Analysis

Despite the evident utility of FISH in patients with AUC results, there is a possibility of false-positive results. Besides "anticipatory positive" FISH results, low specificity and low PPV in some studies might also be due to an increased number of tetraploid or dividing cells under reactive conditions. Although tetraploid cells are not specifically mentioned in the scoring guidelines of the manufacturer, it has now been recognized that rare cells with a tetraploid signal pattern (i.e., four signals of each probe) should not be taken as an unequivocally positive FISH result but interpreted with caution [3, 24–26]. In contrast, unbalanced numerical changes of one or more chromosomes (e.g., 2, 3, 5) or loss of 9p21 is virtually specific for neoplasia in bladder cytology. An exception is that pelvic irradiation (e.g., of the prostate or the uterus) often results in permanent chromosomal aberrations carrying a risk of a false-positive diagnosis by U-FISH. This is particularly the case for polysomies, whereas homozygous or heterozygous deletion of 9p21 remains highly specific for neoplasia even after irradiation. This emphasizes the need of appropriate clinical information and consideration of the typical postirradiation cytological changes. Decoy cells, i.e., polyoma-infected urothelial cells, can easily mislead by a false-positive cytological diagnosis of UC if one is not familiar with the morphological spectrum of decoy cells. Although there have been reports on rare FISH-positive decoy cells, most data suggest that polyomavirus infection does not interfere with U-FISH results [27].

Target FISH, in which there is cytological pre-screening of slides and cells in question prior to FISH, has been proposed as another way of making the FISH analysis more precise and specific by avoiding the analysis of obviously reactive bystander cells or the analysis of remaining material that might be devoid of the atypical cells and therefore not representative of the original slide [6, 24, 25]. This approach requires hybridization and scoring of the original stained slides and automated re-localization of the cells in question, ideally coupled with image-aided interpretation.

Fig. 9.5 (continued) bladder (bladder washing). Highly increased number of all FISH signals due to repeated doubling of the genome (i.e., endoreplication), but no unbalanced copy number changes and no 9p21 deletion. (**b**) Sheets of mildly atypical urothelial cells in a washing of the renal pelvis. Normal FISH result (two copies per chromosome), consistent with reactive changes. (**c**) Atypical urothelial cells suspicious of high grade urothelial carcinoma (SHGUC) in a washing of the renal pelvis. Positive U-FISH result with increased copy numbers of all 3 chromosomes and a homozygous deletion of 9p21. Note the normal cell nucleus with retained 9p21 signals as internal normal control (*right lower corner*). (**d**) U-FISH-positive atypical urothelial cells (SHGUC) with increased copy number of all five chromosomes but no 9p21 deletion. Note the normal cell nucleus with normal copy numbers (*right lower corner*)

ImmunoCyt/uCyt+ and Other Cell-Based Tests

Several cytology-based tests other than DNA in situ hybridization have been developed to improve diagnostic accuracy of urinary cytology, especially its negative predictive value. To put the role of such markers into the right perspective, the performance of cytology is only low for LGUC but not for HGUC. Therefore, combining results of these tests is misleading.

Some of the tests have been approved for diagnostic use and surveillance by the FDA but none of them has been incorporated into recommended guidelines or clinical management [1, 28, 29]. Multiple studies have demonstrated that some urine markers are more sensitive than conventional urine cytology and there is also evidence that these tests may predict tumor progression and risk-stratify patients who are being treated with intravesical therapies [1, 28–32]. Data from meta-analyses suggest that cell-based assays may be more sensitive if compared to other assays especially in low grade tumors [29, 32]. This observation may be explained by the fact that current cell-based assays include markers for low grade tumors and are less confounded by urinary tract infections than liquid-based markers.

ImmunoCyt/uCyt+ Test

The uCyt test developed in 1997 [33] obtained FDA clearance in 2000 for the diagnosis and monitoring of bladder cancer. It combines three fluorescent monoclonal antibodies. Two of them (M344 and LDQ10), labelled with fluorescein (green fluorescence), have been raised against mucin-like antigens. The third one (19A211), labelled with Texas red (red fluorescence), recognizes a high molecular form of carcinoembryonic antigen. An example of a uCyt positive cytological specimen is shown in Fig. 9.6. The uCyt assay is technically simple and less expensive

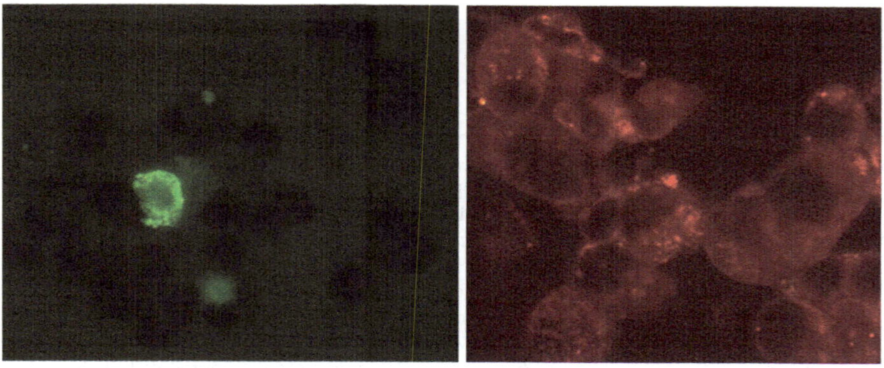

Fig. 9.6 Example of an ImmunoCyt/uCyt+ positive cytological specimen. Positive cells by *red* and *green* immunofluorescence (*Texas red and fluorescein*)

compared with U-FISH methodology and more sensitive in detecting low grade tumors [30]. Slides are read using an epifluorescent microscope with a dual-band filter specific to both fluorescein and Texas Red emission and excitation spectra. Samples are considered positive when at least one green or red fluorescent urothelial cell is observed. The antigens detected by M344 and 19A211 antibodies are expressed by 71 % and 90 % of Ta–T1 bladder tumors, respectively [34]. The usefulness of uCyt has been reported [28–31, 35–38] to detect both low grade and high grade cancers, including in situ carcinoma, as well as to predict recurrence in patients, all with a negative cystoscopy. This has been confirmed in an extensive meta-analysis [32]. The test may have a false-positive result due to inflammatory changes after BCG treatment but its overall sensitivity is high, ranging from 53 to 100 % (average 90 %), especially when combined with cytology (close to 100 %). Sensitivity increases with grade and level of invasion but its specificity is moderate to high (64–95 %; average: 74 %). uCyt improves the sensitivity and negative predictive value in detecting small, low grade tumors which makes this test well-suited for monitoring programs to decrease the frequency of follow-up cystoscopy [30]. However, despite being very promising, the test still needs to be validated in an independent large-scale prospective and multicenter study. Studies on cost-effectiveness are scarce [39].

Other Cell-Based Tests

The ProEx C assay is another promising test consisting of a cocktail of antibodies, which detect both minichromosome maintenance protein (MCM2) and topoisomerase II-alpha protein (TOP2A) and in addition may help to stratify urine specimens difficult to classify morphologically [40, 41]. Other cytologic-based tests have been developed using single antibodies (Ki67, DD23), antibodies against Lewis X antigen, cytokeratin 20, or p16/Ki-67 dual-labelling [42]. A quantitative karyometric cytology system measuring nuclear shape and DNA content in light microscopic images has had variable results in terms of sensitivity and specificity [43]. Of note, almost all tumor markers previously mentioned have a much better sensitivity than cytologic examination but few reach the same level of specificity, and currently are not suitable for the clinical laboratory because of costs.

Liquid-Based Tests

Liquid- or non-cytology-based tests can be applied to voided urine samples either without the need for further preparation or on sediments of centrifuged urine samples. The two most commonly applied liquid-based urine tests on pure voided urine samples are the BTA™ (Polymedco Inc., Cortlandt Manor, NY, USA) and the

NMP22™ (Bladder Check) test (Alere Inc., Waltham, MA, USA), both approved by the FDA, both for detection of bladder cancer in symptomatic patients and for monitoring of patients with a history of bladder cancer. For both tests a qualitative point of care test (BTA stat™ and NMP22-BladderChek™) and a quantitative version (NMP22™ and BTA TRAK™) are available. The latter tests require a dedicated laboratory with specialized personnel. The advantage of a point of care test is that it gives an immediate result and therefore can be done immediately prior to cystoscopy. A positive urine test may lead to a diagnostic review bias, which means that with the knowledge of a positive urine test result, the urologist may be more likely to detect a bladder neoplasm at cystoscopy [44]. These tests have been developed for both voided urine samples (not first-morning urine) and catheter-collected urines but not for barbotage fluids.

BTA Test

The BTA test measures the presence of human complement factor H and related protein, which was shown to be elevated in urine samples of patients with bladder cancer [45]. In this test system the signal is decreased by the presence of factor H-like protein-1, an alternatively spliced product of the complement factor H. Thus, outcome of the BTA™ immunoassay depends on the combined positive and negative signals of the two proteins in a urine sample [46]. For the BTA™ test the urine should be collected without preservatives or fixatives in a clean urine cup and labelled appropriately. The overall sensitivity and specificity of the qualitative point of care BTA™ stat test is 57–83 % and 60–92 %, respectively [47]. The specificity of the BTA™ tests may be overrated by some studies by their exclusion of patients with urinary bladder infection, renal, or bladder stones. The sensitivity of the quantitative BTA TRAK™ test ranges from 62 to 91 % when a cut-off of 14 U/mL is applied. A systematic review [48] demonstrated how bladder cancer patient selection may influence in particular the sensitivity of studied biomarkers. It was shown that the BTA stat™ test had a 12 % lower sensitivity when studies included in the review were restricted to only those with patients under surveillance (sensitivity 58 %) as compared to reviews lacking this selection criterion (70 %). For the BTA TRAK™ test the sensitivity was not much influenced by this selection (sensitivity 71 % and 69 %, respectively). The specificity of the BTA stat™ and BTA TRAK™ test was almost similar in patients under surveillance (73 % for BTA stat™ and 66 % for BTA TRAK™) and in unselected populations (75 % for BTA stat™ and 65 % for BTA TRAK™). In healthy persons without genitourinary signs or symptoms, the specificity of BTAstat is 97 %, but in patients with benign genitourinary conditions the specificity is only 46 % [49]. Any non-neoplastic condition causing hematuria may result in a false-positive BTA™ test, because complement factor H is a normal blood component [50]. The fact that many patients have treatment-related hematuria after intravesical chemo- or immunotherapy without residual or recurrent cancer appears as a limitation of these tests. The BTA stat™ and BTA TRAK™ tests are approved by the FDA to detect bladder cancer in symptomatic patients and for surveillance of patients with bladder cancer.

The NMP22 Test

The NMP22™ test is an immunoassay for the detection of nuclear mitotic apparatus protein [51]. The protein is involved in the distribution of the chromatin to offspring cells, and it is located in the nuclear matrix of all cell types. Its level may correspond to the cellularity and cell turnover in the bladder, rather than a tumor-specific protein [52]. The test should not be performed on samples obtained within 5 days after an invasive procedure as the latter may evoke wound repair potentially leading to a false-positive result. The urine sample needs to be stabilized immediately after collection and it can then be stored at room temperature for 4 days.

The original ELISA-based quantitative assay showed a wide range in sensitivity (47–100 %) and specificity (60–90 %), which is in part influenced by the choice of the cut-off value. Its high false-positive rate due to instrumentation, inflammatory, and regenerative urinary bladder processes reduced its application. For the point of care NMP22 BladderChek™ test a median sensitivity of 50 % and specificity of 87 % was reported [53]. A multi-institutional trial provided evidence for an increased sensitivity of the NMP22 BladderChek™ point of care test over cytology in the detection of bladder cancer in symptomatic patients [54], but the sensitivity of cytology in this study was comparatively poor (17 % for noninvasive and 22 % for invasive carcinomas). Nevertheless, specificity of cytology was better than the NMP22™ test.

A prospective analysis comparing the performance of four commercially available urinary marker tests, including Hemoglobin Dipstick, BTA stat™, NMP22 BladderChek™ and Immunocyt/uCyt+®, the highest sensitivity (94 %) and specificity (84 %) for high grade UC detection was found for the combination of cytology and NMP22 BladderChek™ [55]. In a recently published prospective trial on the cost-effectiveness of the incorporation of NMP22™ and UroVysion® FISH, cystoscopy remained the most cost-effective strategy to detect recurrences of non-muscle invasive bladder cancers, while the addition of urinary markers added to the costs without improving the detection of invasive cancer [56]. Both the quantitative NMP22™ Bladder Cancer ELISA Test Kit and the point of care NMP22 BladderChek™ test are FDA approved for the detection and surveillance of UC in urine samples.

Other Liquid-Based Biomarkers

Urinary biomarkers studying microsatellite instability (loss of heterozygosity), profiling of single nucleotide polymorphisms, DNA methylation, activation of *FGFR3* gene, and gene expression signatures (miRNA) from cellular-extracted nucleic acids have shown some promising results [57]. For example, *FGFR3* mutation analysis in combination with a panel of DNA methylation markers on voided urine could be used to detect recurrences of patients with FGFR3 mutant low grade non-muscle-invasive bladder cancer with a reported sensitivity of 79 % and specificity of 77 % [58]. Also the combination of a panel of different protein markers may increase the sensitivity and specificity of the test [59, 60]. However, further investigation of these biomarkers is needed, preferably in a prospective trial design, before they can be considered for diagnostic use.

Conclusions

The existing evidence strongly points towards a utility of UroVysion® FISH in the setting of atypical urinary cytology. Immunocyt/uCyt+® appears as another promising cell-based test but suffers from limited specificity and needs more validation in cases diagnosed as atypical urinary cytology. Since the definition of "atypia" and its boundaries with "suspicious" have been variable in the past, further studies are needed to better determine the performance of UroVysion® FISH and other ancillary tests in the more stringently and precisely defined "atypical urothelial cells" (AUC) and "suspicious for high grade urothelial carcinoma" (SHGUC) categories of The Paris System. Other urine-based biomarkers for diagnosis and follow-up of UC have little value for the time being and many require further validation.

Liquid-based tests done outside of the cytology laboratory such as BTA- and NMP22-tests have a sensitivity comparable to that of cytology for high grade tumors and are superior for the clinically less important low grade tumors. The International Consultation on Urological Diseases (2012) states that urine marker-guided follow-up of patients with bladder cancer appears feasible, but studies proving the efficacy of this concept and demonstrating an added value for patients or the health system are lacking. Therefore, based on current levels of evidence, systematic marker-guided follow-up cannot be recommended [1]. Until there are new international consensus recommendations on ancillary testing in urinary cytology, U-FISH or Immunocyt/uCyt+® should best be used judiciously on the basis of cytological findings in an individual case after prior consultation with the treating physicians.

Sample Reports UroVysion FISH

Example 1 (AUC, FISH Negative) Renal pelvis (washing): Several clusters of atypical urothelial cells of unknown significance.

The Paris System diagnosis: AUC

Results of UroVysion FISH Testing (Chromosomes 3, 7, 17, and 9p21): Negative

Final diagnosis (cytology & FISH): No evidence of HGUC.

Note: the absence of chromosomal aberrations is in favor of reactive urothelial changes.

However, a low grade urothelial lesion cannot be excluded with certainty, since 20–30 % of these neoplasms are negative by this FISH test.

Example 2 (SHGUC after BCG, FISH Positive) Bladder (washing): Numerous atypical urothelial cells, suspicious of high grade UC.

The Paris System diagnosis: SHGUC

Results of UroVysion FISH Testing (Chromosomes 3, 7, 17, and 9p21): Positive (22/25 cells)

Final diagnosis (cytology & FISH): HGUC.

Note: Almost all atypical cells that were scored revealed pronounced chromosomal aberrations including unbalanced polysomy of the chromosomes 3, 7, and 17, and a relative loss of 9p21. This positive result confirms a diagnosis of high grade UC (at least carcinoma in situ*).*

Example 3 (NHGUC in bladder washing from negative surveillance cystoscopy, FISH positive) Bladder (washing): Monotonous population of mildly atypical cells, cannot exclude LGUN

The Paris System diagnosis: NHGUC; cellular changes suggest LGUN

Results of UroVysion FISH Testing (Chromosomes 3, 7, 17, and 9p21): Positive (18/25 cells)

Final diagnosis (cytology & FISH): Consistent with low grade urothelial neoplasm (LGUN)

Note: The majority of atypical cells that were scored revealed chromosomal aberrations including polysomy of the chromosomes 3, 7, and 17 (3–4 signals instead of 2 signals per chromosome), and a loss of 9p21 (1–2 signals). This positive test result is consistent with a LGUN.

Example 4 (AUC in voided urine, FISH positive) Voided urine: Several degenerated urothelial cells with nuclear atypia of uncertain significance

The Paris System: AUC

Results of UroVysion FISH Testing (Chromosomes 3, 7, 17, and 9p21): Positive (10/25 cells)

Final diagnosis (cytology & FISH): Consistent with urothelial neoplasia (see note)

Note: 10 of the 25 atypical cells that were scored revealed unequivocal chromosomal aberrations including polysomy of chromosomes 3 and 17, and homozygous deletion of 9p21. This positive test result is in favor of urothelial neoplasia. A distinction between low grade and high grade lesion is not possible. We advise further investigations.

Example 5 (NHGUC in bladder washing, tetraploid FISH pattern) Bladder washing: Several urothelial cells with nucelar abnormalities of unknown significance, favor reactive changes.

The Paris System: NHGUC

Results of UroVysion FISH Testing (Chromosomes 3, 7, 17, and 9p21):

Several urothelial cells with a tetraploid chromosomal pattern (6/25)

Final diagnosis (cytology & FISH): No evidence of HGUC (see note).

Note: FISH analysis revealed several cells with a tetraploid pattern (four instead of two signals of each chromosome) but no other abnormalities. Rare tetraploid cells are often found in reactive conditions and are unlikely to point towards urothelial neoplasia. This test result is consistent with reactive urothelial changes.

Appendix

UroVysion® Assay

The slide pretreatment with protease uncovers target DNA and is recommended in Pap-stained specimens. Decolorization is not mandatory since the stain is removed during further phases of FISH procedure. If using the archival slides, remove the coverslip and mounting medium in xylene. Place the slides in 1 % acid alcohol (HCL and 70 % alcohol) overnight or until decolorized. The U-FISH assay can subsequently be conducted either manually or automatically. The first step is denaturation of specimen DNA to expose single-strand target DNA. U-FISH probes should be prepared accordingly and applied to the selected area of slide. The area should be coverslipped and sealed immediately to ensure optimal conditions. Hybridization of probes to target DNA sequences follows under appropriate conditions. The procedure is finished with posthybridization washes to remove excessive probes. Slides should be dried in a dark area. The exact procedure of the FISH assay is described in the UroVysion kit datasheet. The procedure should be validated in each individual laboratory, together with positive and negative controls, to ensure optimal hybridization. Afterwards the specimen chosen for analysis is stained by DAPI solution. Slides are coverslipped and stored at −20 °C in the dark until analysis.

Automated Imaging Systems for UroVysion® FISH Analysis

The Duet TM System™ workstation integrates a microscope, CCD camera, motorized stage or slide-loader, computer, keyboard, mouse, joystick, monitor, and a dedicated software program. Up to 200 slides that have undergone the FISH procedure, can be loaded and run overnight for inspection the following day. This latter feature may be suitable for diagnostic laboratories that receive high volumes of abnormal or atypical urines. Similarly, the Ikoniscope oncoFISH Bladder Test System has an automated scanning microscope system coupled with an image analysis work station. It features automated slide loading and handling, low and high magnification scanning to identify cells of interest, and digital image acquisition [4]. The MetaSystems uses an automated fluorescent scanning microscope and analysis software with "tile-sampling" method [9].

The Bioview Duet System™ scans cells that are imaged at high resolution (under oil immersion) both in bright light illumination and in fluorescent illumination. Cells are classified by the system according to their morphological features, their staining on bright field (Giemsa or Papanicolaou stains, if target FISH is used), and according to the pattern of fluorescent signals. The automated microscope has micrometer-level precision in the X, Y, and Z axes which allows it to focus on cells and retain coordinate information for target cells. There are two modes of operation:

(1) automatic scanning, which provides a gallery of all fields of view, and (2) manual scanning, which provides interactive control allowing the user to select the fields of view using either bright field or fluorescent illumination.

Similar to manual scoring, the automated system scans the FISH slides by locating and scoring the nuclei exhibiting abnormalities such as enlargement, irregular borders, and patchy DAPI staining. As identification of abnormal or malignant cells based solely on aberrant morphology may be misleading, the Bioview System™ classifies cells both by morphology on the DAPI fluorescence, as well as by superimposed FISH signals. Cells are ranked based on a combination of nuclear features, including size, shape, DAPI intensity, and DAPI standard deviation inside the nucleus.

References

1. Kamat AM, Hegarty PK, Gee JR, Clark PE, Svatek RS, Hegarty N, et al. ICUD-EAU International Consultation on Bladder Cancer 2012: screening, diagnosis, and molecular markers. Eur Urol. 2013;63:4–15.
2. Bubendorf L, Piaton E. UroVysion(R) multiprobe FISH in the triage of equivocal urinary cytology cases. Ann Pathol. 2012;32:e52–6. 438–43. [article in French].
3. Halling KC, Kipp BR. Bladder cancer detection using FISH (UroVysion assay). Adv Anat Pathol. 2008;15:279–86.
4. Marganski WA, El-Sirgany Costa V, Kilpatrick MW, Tafas T, Yim J, Matthews M. Digitized microscopy in the diagnosis of bladder cancer: analysis of >3000 cases during a 7-month period. Cancer Cytopathol. 2011;119:279–89.
5. Smith GD, Riding M, Oswald K, Bentz JS. Integrating a FISH imaging system into the cytology laboratory. Cytojournal. 2010;7:3.
6. Smith GD, Bentz JS. "FISHing" to detect urinary and other cancers: validation of an imaging system to aid in interpretation. Cancer Cytopathol. 2010;118:56–64.
7. Daniely M, Rona R, Kaplan T, Olsfanger S, Elboim L, Zilberstien Y, et al. Combined analysis of morphology and fluorescence in situ hybridization significantly increases accuracy of bladder cancer detection in voided urine samples. Urology. 2005;66:1354–9.
8. Bubendorf L. Multiprobe fluorescence in situ hybridization (UroVysion) for the detection of urothelial carcinoma - FISHing for the right catch. Acta Cytol. 2011;55:113–9.
9. Furrer D, Jacob S, Caron C, Sanschagrin F, Provencher L, Diorio C. Validation of a new classifier for the automated analysis of the human epidermal growth factor receptor 2 (HER2) gene amplification in breast cancer specimens. Diagn Pathol. 2013;8:17.
10. Hajdinjak T. UroVysion FISH test for detecting urothelial cancers: meta-analysis of diagnostic accuracy and comparison with urinary cytology testing. Urol Oncol. 2008;26:646–51.
11. Kipp BR, Halling KC, Campion MB, Wendel AJ, Karnes RJ, Zhang J, et al. Assessing the value of reflex fluorescence in situ hybridization testing in the diagnosis of bladder cancer when routine urine cytological examination is equivocal. J Urol. 2008;179:1296–301. discussion 301.
12. Savic S, Zlobec I, Thalmann GN, Engeler D, Schmauss M, Lehmann K, et al. The prognostic value of cytology and fluorescence in situ hybridization in the follow-up of nonmuscle-invasive bladder cancer after intravesical Bacillus Calmette-Guerin therapy. Int J Cancer. 2009;124:2899–904.
13. Gayed BA, Seideman C, Lotan Y. Cost-effectiveness of fluorescence in situ hybridization in patients with atypical cytology for the detection of urothelial carcinoma. J Urol. 2013;190:1181–6.

14. Lotan Y, Bensalah K, Ruddell T, Shariat SF, Sagalowsky AI, Ashfaq R. Prospective evaluation of the clinical usefulness of reflex fluorescence in situ hybridization assay in patients with atypical cytology for the detection of urothelial carcinoma of the bladder. J Urol. 2008;179:2164–9.
15. Schlomer BJ, Ho R, Sagalowsky A, Ashfaq R, Lotan Y. Prospective validation of the clinical usefulness of reflex fluorescence in situ hybridization assay in patients with atypical cytology for the detection of urothelial carcinoma of the bladder. J Urol. 2010;183:62–7.
16. Kim PH, Sukhu R, Cordon BH, Sfakianos JP, Sjoberg DD, Hakimi AA, et al. Reflex fluorescence in situ hybridization assay for suspicious urinary cytology in patients with bladder cancer with negative surveillance cystoscopy. BJU Int. 2014;114:354–9.
17. Seideman C, Canter D, Kim P, Cordon B, Weizer A, Oliva I, et al. Multicenter evaluation of the role of UroVysion FISH assay in surveillance of patients with bladder cancer: does FISH positivity anticipate recurrence? World J Urol. 2014. doi:10.1007/s00345-014-1452-9. Epub ahead of print.
18. Skacel M, Fahmy M, Brainard JA, Pettay JD, Biscotti CV, Liou LS, et al. Multitarget fluorescence in situ hybridization assay detects transitional cell carcinoma in the majority of patients with bladder cancer and atypical or negative urine cytology. J Urol. 2003;169:2101–5.
19. Yoder BJ, Skacel M, Hedgepeth R, Babineau D, Ulchaker JC, Liou LS, et al. Reflex UroVysion testing of bladder cancer surveillance patients with equivocal or negative urine cytology: a prospective study with focus on the natural history of anticipatory positive findings. Am J Clin Pathol. 2007;127:295–301.
20. Fritsche HM, Burger M, Dietmaier W, Denzinger S, Bach E, Otto W, et al. Multicolor FISH (UroVysion) facilitates follow-up of patients with high-grade urothelial carcinoma of the bladder. Am J Clin Pathol. 2010;134:597–603.
21. Kipp BR, Karnes RJ, Brankley SM, Harwood AR, Pankratz VS, Sebo TJ, et al. Monitoring intravesical therapy for superficial bladder cancer using fluorescence in situ hybridization. J Urol. 2005;173:401–4.
22. Whitson J, Berry A, Carroll P, Konety B. A multicolour fluorescence in situ hybridization test predicts recurrence in patients with high-risk superficial bladder tumours undergoing intravesical therapy. BJU Int. 2009;104:336–9.
23. Mengual L, Marin-Aguilera M, Ribal MJ, Burset M, Villavicencio H, Oliver A, et al. Clinical utility of fluorescent in situ hybridization for the surveillance of bladder cancer patients treated with bacillus Calmette-Guerin therapy. Eur Urol. 2007;52:752–9.
24. Huysentruyt CJ, Baldewijns MM, Ruland AM, Tonk RJ, Vervoort PS, Smits KM, et al. Modified UroVysion scoring criteria increase the urothelial carcinoma detection rate in cases of equivocal urinary cytology. Histopathology. 2011;58:1048–53.
25. Tapia C, Glatz K, Obermann EC, Grilli B, Barascud A, Herzog M, et al. Evaluation of chromosomal aberrations in patients with benign conditions and reactive changes in urinary cytology. Cancer Cytopathol. 2011;119:404–10.
26. Zellweger T, Benz G, Cathomas G, Mihatsch MJ, Sulser T, Gasser TC, et al. Multi-target fluorescence in situ hybridization in bladder washings for prediction of recurrent bladder cancer. Int J Cancer. 2006;119:1660–5.
27. Hossain D, Hull D, Kalantarpour F, Maitlen R, Qian J, Bostwick DG. Does polyomavirus infection interfere with bladder cancer fluorescence in situ hybridization? Diagn Cytopathol. 2014;42:225–9.
28. Kamat AM, Vlahou A, Taylor JA, Hudson ML, Pesch B, Ingersoll MA, et al. Considerations on the use of urine markers in the management of patients with high-grade non-muscle-invasive bladder cancer. Urol Oncol. 2014;32:1069–77.
29. Schmitz-Drager BJ, Todenhofer T, van Rhijn B, Pesch B, Hudson MA, Chandra A, et al. Considerations on the use of urine markers in the management of patients with low-/intermediate-risk non-muscle invasive bladder cancer. Urol Oncol. 2014;32:1061–8.
30. Sullivan PS, Nooraie F, Sanchez H, Hirschowitz S, Levin M, Rao PN, et al. Comparison of ImmunoCyt, UroVysion, and urine cytology in detection of recurrent urothelial carcinoma: a "split-sample" study. Cancer. 2009;117:167–73.

31. Todenhofer T, Hennenlotter J, Esser M, Mohrhardt S, Tews V, Aufderklamm S, et al. Combined application of cytology and molecular urine markers to improve the detection of urothelial carcinoma. Cancer Cytopathol. 2013;121:252–60.
32. Yang M, Zheng Z, Zhuang Z, Zhao X, Xu Z, Lin H. ImmunoCyt and cytology for diagnosis of bladder carcinoma: a meta analysis. Chin Med J (Engl). 2014;127:758–64.
33. Fradet Y, Lockhard C. Performance characteristics of a new monoclonal antibody test for bladder cancer: ImmunoCyt trade mark. Can J Urol. 1997;4:400–5.
34. Allard P, Fradet Y, Tetu B, Bernard P. Tumor-associated antigens as prognostic factors for recurrence in 382 patients with primary transitional cell carcinoma of the bladder. Clin Cancer Res. 1995;1:1195–202.
35. Comploj E, Mian C, Ambrosini-Spaltro A, Dechet C, Palermo S, Trenti E, et al. uCyt+/ImmunoCyt and cytology in the detection of urothelial carcinoma: an update on 7422 analyses. Cancer Cytopathol. 2013;121:392–7.
36. Mian C, Pycha A, Wiener H, Haitel A, Lodde M, Marberger M. Immunocyt: a new tool for detecting transitional cell cancer of the urinary tract. J Urol. 1999;161:1486–9.
37. Piaton E, Daniel L, Verriele V, Dalifard I, Zimmermann U, Renaudin K, et al. Improved detection of urothelial carcinomas with fluorescence immunocytochemistry (uCyt+ assay) and urinary cytology: results of a French Prospective Multicenter Study. Lab Invest. 2003;83:845–52.
38. Tetu B, Tiguert R, Harel F, Fradet Y. ImmunoCyt/uCyt+ improves the sensitivity of urine cytology in patients followed for urothelial carcinoma. Mod Pathol. 2005;18:83–9.
39. Mowatt G, Zhu S, Kilonzo M, Boachie C, Fraser C, Griffiths TR, et al. Systematic review of the clinical effectiveness and cost-effectiveness of photodynamic diagnosis and urine biomarkers (FISH, ImmunoCyt, NMP22) and cytology for the detection and follow-up of bladder cancer. Health Technol Assess. 2010;14:1–331. iii-iv.
40. Moatamed NA, Rao JY, Alexanian S, Cobarrubias M, Levin M, Lu D, et al. ProEx C as an adjunct marker to improve cytological detection of urothelial carcinoma in urinary specimens. Cancer Cytopathol. 2013;121:320–8.
41. Vergara-Lluri ME, Hu E, Rao JY, Levin M, Apple SK, Moatamed NA. Comparative evaluation of ProEx C and ImmunoCyt/uCyt assays in atypical urine cytology. Arch Pathol Lab Med. 2014;138:1215–22.
42. Piaton E, Carre C, Advenier AS, Decaussin-Petrucci M, Mege-Lechevallier F, Lantier P, et al. p16 INK4a overexpression and p16/Ki-67 dual labeling versus conventional urinary cytology in the evaluation of urothelial carcinoma. Cancer Cytopathol. 2014;122:211–20.
43. Tetu B. Diagnosis of urothelial carcinoma from urine. Mod Pathol. 2009;22 Suppl 2:S53–9.
44. van der Aa MN, Steyerberg EW, Bangma C, van Rhijn BW, Zwarthoff EC, van der Kwast TH. Cystoscopy revisited as the gold standard for detecting bladder cancer recurrence: diagnostic review bias in the randomized, prospective CEFUB trial. J Urol. 2010;183:76–80.
45. Kinders R, Jones T, Root R, Bruce C, Murchison H, Corey M, et al. Complement factor H or a related protein is a marker for transitional cell cancer of the bladder. Clin Cancer Res. 1998;4:2511–20.
46. Cheng ZZ, Corey MJ, Parepalo M, Majno S, Hellwage J, Zipfel PF, et al. Complement factor H as a marker for detection of bladder cancer. Clin Chem. 2005;51:856–63.
47. Tilki D, Burger M, Dalbagni G, Grossman HB, Hakenberg OW, Palou J, et al. Urine markers for detection and surveillance of non-muscle-invasive bladder cancer. Eur Urol. 2011;60:484–92.
48. van Rhijn BW, van der Poel HG, van der Kwast TH. Urine markers for bladder cancer surveillance: a systematic review. Eur Urol. 2005;47:736–48.
49. Leyh H, Marberger M, Conort P, Sternberg C, Pansadoro V, Pagano F, et al. Comparison of the BTA stat test with voided urine cytology and bladder wash cytology in the diagnosis and monitoring of bladder cancer. Eur Urol. 1999;35:52–6.
50. Oge O, Kozaci D, Gemalmaz H. The BTA stat test is nonspecific for hematuria: an experimental hematuria model. J Urol. 2002;167:1318–9. discussion 9-20.

51. Soloway MS, Briggman V, Carpinito GA, Chodak GW, Church PA, Lamm DL, et al. Use of a new tumor marker, urinary NMP22, in the detection of occult or rapidly recurring transitional cell carcinoma of the urinary tract following surgical treatment. J Urol. 1996;156(2 Pt 1):363–7.
52. Miyake M, Goodison S, Giacoia EG, Rizwani W, Ross S, Rosser CJ. Influencing factors on the NMP-22 urine assay: an experimental model. BMC Urol. 2012;12:23.
53. Zhou AG, Hutchinson LM, Ceosar EF. Urine cytopathology and ancillary methods. Surg Pathol Clin. 2014;7:77–88.
54. Grossman HB, Messing E, Soloway M, Tomera K, Katz G, Berger Y, et al. Detection of bladder cancer using a point-of-care proteomic assay. JAMA. 2005;293:810–6.
55. Yafi FA, Brimo F, Auger M, Aprikian A, Tanguay S, Kassouf W. Is the performance of urinary cytology as high as reported historically? A contemporary analysis in the detection and surveillance of bladder cancer. Urol Oncol. 2014;32:27. e1-6.
56. Kamat AM, Karam JA, Grossman HB, Kader AK, Munsell M, Dinney CP. Prospective trial to identify optimal bladder cancer surveillance protocol: reducing costs while maximizing sensitivity. BJU Int. 2011;108:1119–23.
57. Sapre N, Anderson PD, Costello AJ, Hovens CM, Corcoran NM. Gene-based urinary biomarkers for bladder cancer: an unfulfilled promise? Urol Oncol. 2014;32:48. e9-17.
58. Zuiverloon TC, van der Aa MN, van der Kwast TH, Steyerberg EW, Lingsma HF, Bangma CH, et al. Fibroblast growth factor receptor 3 mutation analysis on voided urine for surveillance of patients with low-grade non-muscle-invasive bladder cancer. Clin Cancer Res. 2010;16:3011–8.
59. Chen LM, Chang M, Dai Y, Chai KX, Dyrskjot L, Sanchez-Carbayo M, et al. External validation of a multiplex urinary protein panel for the detection of bladder cancer in a multicenter cohort. Cancer Epidemiol. 2014;23:1804–12.
60. Kandimalla R, Masius R, Beukers W, Bangma CH, Orntoft TF, Dyrskjot L, et al. A 3-plex methylation assay combined with the FGFR3 mutation assay sensitively detects recurrent bladder cancer in voided urine. Clin Cancer Res. 2013;19:4760–9.

Chapter 10
Cytopreparatory Techniques

Gary W. Gill, William N. Crabtree, and Deidra P. Kelly

Background

Regardless of the source of cells or reporting system, the role of cytopreparation in the diagnostic process must be recognized and explicitly detailed because cytopreparation can affect the cytomorphological findings at least as much as the underlying biology of the cells or the expertise of the cytologist. Cytopreparation is a combination of methods for optimizing and standardizing the collection, preparation, and analysis of cytologic samples in ways that promote the detection of cells of interest and accurate interpretation of nuclear morphology.

For these reasons, laboratories are wise to invest in the valuable technical skillset known as cytopreparation. The practice of cytopreparation involves the analysis of each step, device, method, and reagents that the cells encounter between removal from the body and morphological analysis at the microscope. Collectively, cytopreparatory techniques that a lab uses for processing a specimen constitute a standard operating procedure, each one with its own applicable terms of cellular preservation, flattening, chromatin distribution and particle size, biochemical makeup, stainability, interaction with light, and cost. Laboratorians must often balance the trade-offs of all the steps required by the device, preparation methods, and reagents in order to arrive at a standard operating procedure that best matches the laboratory's clinical needs and financial constraints.

Materials and Methods

Collection

In terms of cellularity and preservation there is a trade-off between the invasiveness of the clinical procedure and the cellular yield: bladder washings are best, catheterized urines are second, and voided specimens are third. The collection method

D.L. Rosenthal et al. (eds.), *The Paris System for Reporting Urinary Cytology*,
DOI 10.1007/978-3-319-22864-8_10

should not impact the processing method unless the volume of instrumented specimens is artificially high. The impact of collection techniques on adequacy criteria is addressed in Chap. 2.

Processing

- A collection method should harvest well-preserved cells that reliably represent any urinary tract lesion that might be present.
- Use sterile, pyrogen-free balanced salt solutions in bladder instrumentation. Normal saline (i.e., 0.9 % NaCl w/v) is discouraged [1] as it may ruin cell morphology [2].
- As urine itself may degrade cells that have been sitting in the bladder for extended periods of time, cells expelled during the first void of the morning are less than optimal; it is best to discard the initial voided urine, and use the next voided fresh urine after the patient drinks 8–16 oz of water.
- In the laboratory, if the specimens appear turbid, add acetic acid a few drops at a time, vortex. If cloudiness persists, repeat until clarity results [3].
- Ideally freshly collected urine specimens should be processed promptly after collection. Cells in urine specimens may be degenerated at the time of collection, and no amount of preservative can save them and may even increase cellular degeneration [4].
- Process urine specimens within about 4 h, and if this is not feasible, specimens may be refrigerated for up to 12 h without noticeable effects on quality. However, refrigeration accelerates the precipitation of salts in urines.
- Historically, some protocols have used a microscopic inspection of a drop of *unstained* specimen in order to determine the optimal input of resuspended supernatant. This is rarely if ever done in modern laboratories but may prove useful in certain challenging specimens if a first slide prepared with a standard automated technique is unsatisfactory.

Preparation Methods

Following good principles and practices of cytopreparation, all processing methods will produce satisfactory results [3]. This is shown by Figs. 10.1, 10.2, 10.3, and10.4 showing different urine specimens processed by membrane filtration (e.g., Millipore), cytocentrifugation (i.e., Shandon Cytospin), (CS), and the liquid-based preparations, BD SurePath Prep (SP), and Hologic ThinPrep (TP).

Millipore Filtration **(EMD Millipore, Billerica, MA)**
The specimen is collected fresh (i.e., without added alcohol as a preservative), and concentrated by conventional centrifugation. The supernatant was discarded, and the cell button was resuspended by being vortexed in a few mL of balanced electrolyte solution. The resuspended cells were processed by membrane filtration

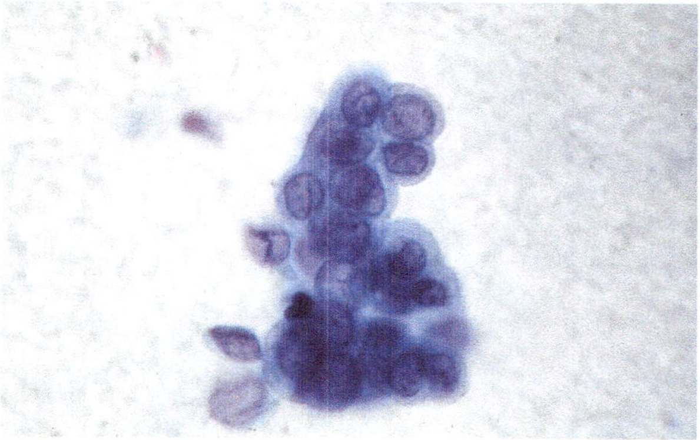

Fig. 10.1 Low grade urothelial neoplasia (*Voided fresh urine, Millipore filtration, high mag.*)

Fig. 10.2 Low grade urothelial neoplasia (*Voided fresh urine, CS, high mag.*)

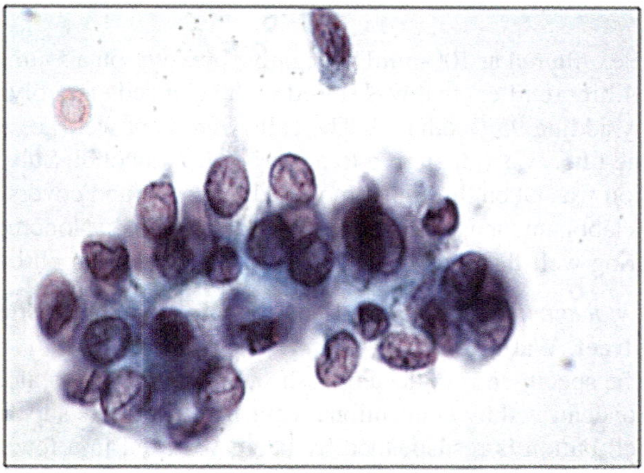

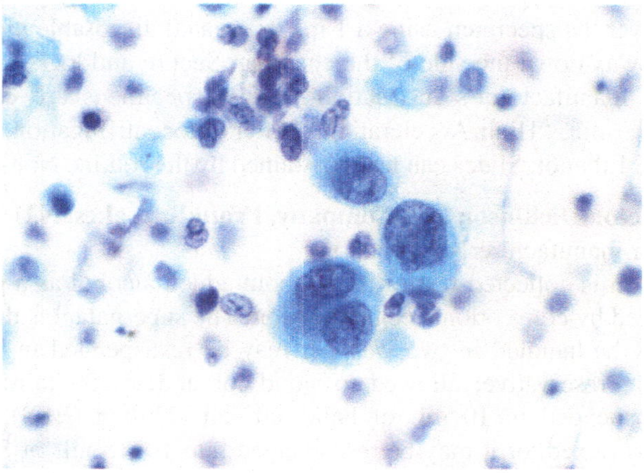

Fig. 10.3 Atypical urothelial cells (*Voided fresh urine, SP, high mag.*)

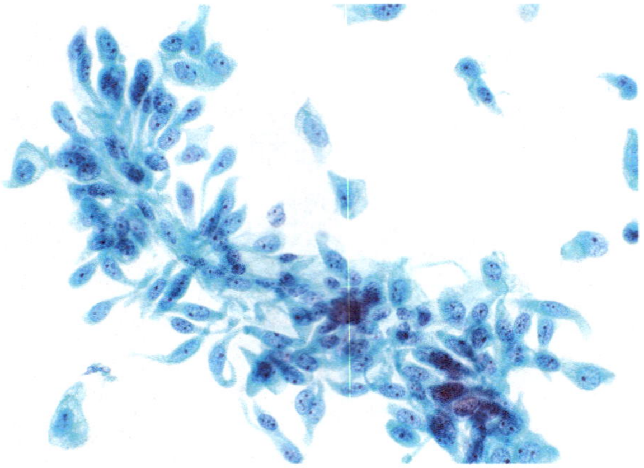

Fig. 10.4 Cercariaform urothelial cells from a case of LGUN *(Voided urine, TP, high mag.)*

(i.e., filtered at 100-mmHg negative pressure on a 5-μm pore size, 47-mm-diameter Millipore filter) that was rinsed with balanced electrolyte solution, and fixed in situ by adding 95 % ethanol. The cells were kept wet (i.e., not allowed to air-dry), and the filter was transferred to a Petri dish of alcohol. Subsequently, the filter preparation was taken through a modified Pap stain and coverslipped. Membrane filtration is labor-intensive, and is rarely used these days. Nonetheless, it is capable of recovering well-flattened cells that display their nuclear chromatin usefully.

Cytocentrifugation **(Shandon Cytospin, Thermo Fisher Scientific, 81 Wyman Street, Waltham, MA)**
The specimen is collected fresh (i.e., without added alcohol as a preservative), and concentrated by conventional centrifugation. The supernatant is discarded, and the cell button is resuspended by being vortexed in a few mL of balanced electrolyte solution. Place the specimen volume in the sample chamber (DO NOT EXCEED 0.25 mL) using a 1 mL graduated disposable pipette. Carefully layer 0.25 mL of 2 % carbowax over the specimen using a 1 mL graduated disposable pipette by dripping the carbowax down the side of the chamber. Secure and lock the chamber in place per the manufacturer's instructions. Urine specimens are centrifuged at 1000 rpm for 8 min, "High Acceleration." After cytocentrifugation, immediately wet fix in 95 % Ethanol. Slides can be Pap-stained by the routine Non-Gyn method.

SurePath® **(Becton Dickinson and Company, Franklin Lakes, NJ)**
Preparation per manufacturer's instructions.

The specimen is collected fresh (i.e., without added alcohol as a preservative), and concentrated by conventional centrifugation. The supernatant is discarded. The cell pellet may be handled in two ways. It may be resuspended in 10–15 mL of CytoRich Red Preservative; allowed to stand for at least 30 min; centrifuged; decanted; resuspended in 10 mL of balanced salt solution (BSS); centrifuged; decanted and vortexed, or it may be resuspended into 10–15 mL of SurePath Gyn

Preservative Fluid or CytoRich Clear Preservative; vortexed; allowed to stand for at least 30 min; centrifuged; decanted and vortexed. The pelleted cells are then placed on the SurePath PrepStain device where they are resuspended, mixed, and transferred to a PrepStain Settling Chamber mounted on a SurePath PreCoat slide. The cells are sedimented by gravity, then stained using a modified Papanicolaou staining procedure. The slide is cleared in xylene or a xylene substitute and coverslipped. The cells are presented within a 13-mm-diameter circle

ThinPrep® **(Hologic, Bedford, MA)**
Preparation per manufacturer's instructions.

The specimen is collected fresh (i.e., without added alcohol as a preservative), and concentrated by conventional centrifugation. The supernatant is discarded, and the cell button is resuspended with PreservCyt and the sample vial is placed into a ThinPrep 2000 Processor. A gentle dispersion step breaks up blood, mucus, nondiagnostic debris, and thoroughly mixes the cell sample. The cells are then collected on a ThinPrep Filter specifically designed to collect diagnostic cells. The ThinPrep 2000 Processor constantly monitors the rate of flow through the ThinPrep Filter during the collection process in order to prevent the cellular presentation from being too scant or too dense. A thin layer of cells is then transferred to a glass slide in a 20-mm-diameter circle, and the slide is automatically deposited into a fixative solution. Routine Papanicolaou staining method finalizes the process.

Discussion

A cursory review of the scientific literature reveals no generally accepted best materials and methods of collecting and processing urine to detect urothelial malignancies. Various citations come to different conclusions about the pros and cons of urine that is voided spontaneously vs. catheterized vs. bladder washings [5], as well as number of urine specimens [6], whether urine should be collected fresh or preserved [4], whether to keep at room temperature or refrigerate [4–6], how many hours, the number of urine specimens needed to improve sensitivity [7], which processing method is best [8–10], and the number of cells to define adequacy [11, 12]. Some basic principles appear to have broad consensus and are compatible with common sense.

Conclusions and Recommendations

Cytology terminology reporting systems are essential to good patient management, and good cytopreparatory techniques are essential to producing cells suitable for being described by standardized terminology reporting systems. The word "technique" is deliberately chosen, as it means a particular way of doing something—compared to another similar-appearing way—that makes a useful difference.

The urine collection and processing guidance in this chapter must be followed by consistently good staining and mounting techniques for best results. Readers are referred elsewhere for that guidance [3, 13, 14].

References

1. Awad S, Allison SP, Lobo DN. The history of 0.9% saline. Clin Nutr. 2008;27:179–88.
2. Pomerat CM, Overman RR. Electrolytes and plasma expanders – I. Reaction of human cells in perfusion chambers with phase contrast, time-lapse cine records. Z Zellforsch Mikrosk Anat. 1956;45:2–17.
3. Gill GW. Cytopreparation: principles & practice. In: Rosenthal DL, series editor. Essentials in cytopathology, Vol. 12. New York: Springer; 2013
4. Crabtree WN, Murphy WM. The value of ethanol as a fixative in urinary cytology. Acta Cytol. 1980;24:452–5.
5. Murphy WM. Current status of urinary cytology in the evaluation of bladder neoplasms. Hum Pathol. 1990;21:886–96.
6. Murphy WM, Crabtree WN, Jukkola AF, Soloway MS. The diagnostic value of urine versus bladder washing in patients with bladder cancer. J Urol. 1981;126:320–2.
7. Beyer-Boon ME, de Voogt HJ, van der Velde EA, Brussee JA, Schaberg A. The efficacy of urinary cytology in the detection of urothelial tumours. Sensitivity and specificity of urinary cytology. Urol Res. 1978;6:3–12.
8. Beyer-Boon ME, Voorn-den Hollander MJ. Cell yield obtained with various cytopreparatory techniques for urinary cytology. Acta Cytol. 1978;22:589–93.
9. Beyer-Boon ME, van der Voorn-Den Hollander MJ, Arentz PW, Cornelisse CJ, Schaberg A, Fox CH. Effect of various routine cytopreparatory techniques on normal urothelial cells and their nuclei. Acta Pathol Microbiol Scand A. 1979;87:63–9.
10. Voss JS, Kipp BR, Krueger AK, Clayton AC, Halling KC, Karnes RJ, et al. Changes in specimen preparation method may impact urine cytologic evaluation. Am J Clin Pathol. 2008;130:428–33.
11. Hundley AF, Maygarden S, Wu JM, Visco AG, Connolly A. Adequacy of urine cytology specimens: an assessment of collection techniques. Int Urogynecol J Pelvic Floor Dysfunct. 2007;18:997–1001.
12. Prather J, Arville B, Chatt G, Pambuccian SE, Wojcik EM, Quek ML, Barkan GA. Evidence-based adequacy criteria for urinary bladder barbotage cytology. J Am Soc Cytol. 2015;4:57–62.
13. Gill GW. Chapter 28: The laboratory. In: DeMay RM, editor. The Art & science of cytopathology, vol. 3. 2nd ed. Chicago: ASCP Press; 2011. p. 1539–92.
14. Gill GW. Chapter 6: Fixation and specimen processing. In: Gupta PK, Baloch ZW, editors. Cytohistology of small tissue samples. New York: Cambridge University Press; 2011. p. 148–61.

Chapter 11
Clinical Management

Marcus L. Quek, Trinity J. Bivalacqua, Ashish M. Kamat, and Mark P. Schoenberg

Background

Urine cytology remains an important adjunctive test in the diagnostic armamentarium of the urologist. The utility of cytology is dependent on several factors including the disease process, the adequacy of the specimen collection, and especially the skill of the cytopathologist. As such, the clinician must understand and appreciate the inherent limitations of cytology. Standardization of the diagnostic criteria and reporting system has long been sought after to aid in clinical decision-making and comparative study. The Paris System for Reporting Urine Cytology (The Paris System) provides the basis for a common language for both cytopathologists and the clinician.

The clinical scenarios in which urine cytology are performed include the evaluation of hematuria and voiding symptoms, initial workup for a suspected urothelial malignancy, and for surveillance following treatment for urothelial cancer. The decision to obtain a voided or instrumented (barbotage/washing/brushing) cytology depends on the clinical setting. Herein, we review the clinical management for each of the diagnostic categories of The Paris System.

Management of Negative for High Grade Urothelial Carcinoma (NHGUC)

Urine cytology has always demonstrated accuracy in detecting high grade tumors and carcinoma in situ (CIS) [1, 2]. Mortality from bladder cancer is overwhelmingly due to these lesions. The designation of "Negative for High Grade Urothelial Carcinoma" (NHGUC) as a distinct diagnostic category highlights the utility of cytology in identifying these potentially dangerous lesions within

D.L. Rosenthal et al. (eds.), *The Paris System for Reporting Urinary Cytology*,
DOI 10.1007/978-3-319-22864-8_11

the urinary tract. It also acknowledges the inherent limitations of cytology in detecting low grade noninvasive cancers which represent the majority of bladder cancer diagnoses. It is therefore not surprising that the overall sensitivity for cytology to detect bladder cancer is low [1]. The acceptance of standardized criteria for this category will have the resulting beneficial effect of decreasing the number of specimens allocated to the "wastebasket" diagnostic category of "atypical urothelial cells."

The primary concern is whether there is a "clinically significant" lesion somewhere in the urinary tract. From the standpoint of the urologist and especially the patient, the first question is whether there is a malignancy, and secondly, whether that cancer is potentially lethal. While cytology may not perform well in answering the first question (due to the poor sensitivity to detect low grade noninvasive tumors), its ability to provide insight into the second question can be very useful depending on the clinical setting.

The role of urine cytology in the initial evaluation for hematuria or irritative voiding symptoms is controversial. In fact, the American Urological Association guidelines on asymptomatic microhematuria do not recommend the use of cytology in the routine evaluation of the asymptomatic microhematuria patient [3]. The Guidelines leave open the *option* for urine cytology only for those with persistent microhematuria following a negative evaluation or those with risk factors for carcinoma in situ (CIS) (irritative voiding symptoms, current or previous tobacco use, chemical exposures). In the setting of a patient with no previous urothelial malignancy, a negative urine cytology result is certainly reassuring, though should not preclude an otherwise thorough urologic evaluation if the clinical scenario calls for it, which generally should include upper tract imaging and direct cystoscopic visualization.

For the patient undergoing the initial evaluation for a suspected urothelial malignancy, urine cytology may play an important role in risk stratification [4]. The finding of a negative cytology result in the face of an obvious papillary bladder tumor should not come as a surprise given the low sensitivity of cytology for the majority of low grade noninvasive tumors. In this setting, the urologist can be reassured that an underlying high grade invasive lesion or CIS is less likely to be present. A positive cytology without a tumor should raise suspicion of a missed lesion and/or missed CIS, for which adjuncts to regular cystoscopy (such as fluorescence cystoscopy, narrow band imaging, and directed or random biopsies of the bladder) and evaluation of the prostatic urethra and upper tracts should be considered.

Urine cytology plays a critical role in the ongoing surveillance for urothelial recurrences following therapy. While most bladder recurrences will often be detected by routine surveillance cystoscopy, upper urinary tract and prostatic or urethral recurrences can be more difficult to diagnose in a timely manner. Anterior bladder wall and bladder neck lesions can occasionally be missed, while carcinoma in situ may not always be readily distinguishable cystoscopically from other benign inflammatory conditions. Thoughtful utilization of contrast-enhanced imaging along with urine cytology represents the primary initial diagnostic modalities when direct endoscopic visualization can be difficult or impractical.

A variety of surveillance strategies have been advocated following transurethral resection with and without intravesical therapies. The most common approach has included cystoscopic assessment every 3 months in the first 2 years, followed by every 6 months for the subsequent 2–3 years, and then annually thereafter (American Urological Association Guidelines) [4]. The European Association of Urology recommends a risk-adapted approach for surveillance depending on the primary tumor stage and grade and presence of CIS [5]. Urine cytology may be obtained at each follow-up surveillance cystoscopy via voided specimen or bladder barbotage (washing) as the situation dictates.

Urine cytology is also an essential component in the surveillance of patients who undergo urinary diversion, as these patients remain at risk for recurrences in the remnant urothelium (upper tracts and urethra) following radical cystectomy [6–9]. Voided specimens for those with orthotopic neobladders, catheterized specimens from incontinent and continent cutaneous diversions, as well as urethral washings provide important diagnostic information some times before lesions become radiographically or symptomatically evident. Risk factors for urethral and upper tract recurrences following radical cystectomy have previously been described [7–10]. A "negative for high grade urothelial carcinoma" diagnosis is reassuring and the patient may continue routine surveillance at intervals commensurate with the risk of recurrence. It must be noted, however, that cytology in the setting of a urinary diversion requires special attention and skill by the cytopathologist to interpret, and hence imaging and symptom review remain essential parts of the surveillance paradigm.

Management of Atypical Urothelial Cells

The management of "atypical urothelial cells (AUC)" has always presented a diagnostic dilemma for the urologist. Traditionally, this category has included a wide spectrum of benign and malignant conditions. The use of the current reporting system should decrease the rate of AUC diagnoses, as known benign conditions such as reactive/inflammatory conditions and cellular changes associated with polyomavirus and urolithiasis will now be categorized as NHGUC. At this point, it is not entirely clear how this will impact the risk of malignancy associated with an AUC diagnosis. On the one hand, as the number of benign conditions will be shifted to the NHGUC category, some cases of AUC will likely now fall into the category of suspicious for HGUC (SHGUC). In either case, the frequency of AUC should decrease.

From the standpoint of the urologist, the workup for AUC should be individualized based on the risk assessment of the patient. Those with hematuria or persistent irritative voiding symptoms still require a thorough evaluation with upper tract imaging and cystoscopy. A patient with known risk factors for urothelial carcinoma and an atypical cytology should prompt consideration of performing further testing to rule out malignancy. For patients with a prior history of urothelial malignancy, the extent of the workup is dependent on the clinical suspicion for recurrent disease. Evaluation of the upper urinary tract and urethra may be considered if not recently performed. The utility of random bladder biopsies of "normal" appearing urothelium is likely of minimal benefit.

The role of additional molecular testing, such as UroVysion FISH and other urinary biomarkers, remains to be determined [1, 2, 11] (see Chap. 9). Several centers have instituted reflex UroVysion FISH testing for AUC diagnoses, whereby a positive FISH assay is managed similarly to a suspicious diagnosis and a negative FISH test is followed expectantly [12–14]. Further investigation is needed to determine the clinical effectiveness of this protocol in light of The Paris System (see Chap. 9).

Management of Suspicious/Positive for High Grade Urothelial Carcinoma

From a practical standpoint, the clinical management of "suspicious for HGUC" (SHGUC) is similar to a "positive for HGUC" (HGUC) diagnosis. These patients require active investigation in order to identify the source of the suspicious or positive cells. When a "suspicious" or "positive" for HGUC cytology result is obtained in the setting of a low grade noninvasive bladder cancer (LGUC), consideration should strongly be given to further evaluation for other high grade lesions or CIS utilizing adjuncts to regular cystoscopy (fluorescence cystoscopy, narrow band imaging, directed/random bladder biopsies) and evaluation of the prostatic urethra and upper tracts.

Upper tract evaluation with multiphase contrast-enhanced cross-sectional imaging with computerized tomography (CT urography) is considered the current standard imaging modality. For those with contraindications to contrast administration, alternatives may include magnetic resonance urography and renal ultrasound with retrograde pyelography. Any upper tract abnormalities should be further evaluated with direct endoscopic (ureteroscopic) visualization with biopsies of any suspicious areas if feasible. Cystourethroscopy remains the mainstay of evaluation of the lower urinary tract. Biopsies and formal transurethral resection of mucosal abnormalities is indicated. For those with negative upper tract imaging and cystoscopy, selective cytologic sampling from both upper tracts may help further localize lesions such as CIS which may be difficult to visualize radiographically. The role of enhanced direct endoscopic techniques, such as fluorescence ("Blue Light") cystoscopy with 5-aminolevulinic acid (5-ALA) or narrow band imaging may further improve the ability to detect more subtle lesions compared with conventional white-light cystoscopy [15–21].

For the subset of patients being followed post-cystectomy and urinary diversion, a finding of suspicious or positive for HGUC also warrants a thorough investigation. Recurrences in the intestinal segment itself are extremely unlikely. Investigations should focus on the upper tracts as well as the urethra. Prostatic stromal invasion and anterior vaginal wall involvement with urothelial carcinoma portends a high risk for urethral recurrences following cystectomy, especially in those diverted by means of a cutaneous diversion (ileal conduit or continence cutaneous reservoir) [6, 8, 10]. Urethral wash cytologies are sometimes employed in the routine follow-up of these patients (if a prophylactic urethrectomy is not performed) based on the specific risk factors (multifocal CIS, tumors at the bladder neck or prostatic urethra). For those with orthotopic neobladders, a positive/suspicious voided cytology may be further investigated with cystoscopy and biopsies as indicated. Risk factors for upper tract recurrences have previously been reported [7, 9]. Patients with suspected upper tract recurrences following cystectomy and diversion often require direct percutaneous access to the upper tract for antegrade ureterorenoscopy since retrograde access through the ureteroenteric anastamosis may be challenging. Management of lesions identified in the remnant urothelium can be treated via endoscopic resection (antegrade/retrograde), instillation of topical immuno- or chemotherapeutics, and surgical resection depending on the clinical scenario [6].

Management of Low Grade Urothelial Neoplasms

As mentioned previously the ability to diagnose low grade urothelial neoplasms (LGUN) based on cytology can be challenging. The majority of bladder cancers present as low grade noninvasive papillary tumors. While these typically demonstrate a low likelihood of metastasis, recurrences are common. Transurethral resection establishes the histologic diagnosis and is therapeutic for most solitary low grade tumors. A single postoperative instillation of intravesical chemotherapy (such as mitomycin C) has shown some benefit in decreasing the frequency of recurrences [4]. Routine surveillance cystoscopies may be performed in the office at regular intervals. The European Association of Urology recommends a risk-adapted surveillance protocol for non-muscle-invasive bladder cancer [5]. The decision to give adjuvant intravesical therapy (chemotherapy or immunotherapy) is based on the risk of recurrence and progression [22]. The indications include large tumors, tumor multifocality, presence of CIS, any high grade component, invasion into the lamina propria, and prior tumor recurrences [4]. Various agents have been utilized including cytotoxic chemotherapy (mitomycin, doxorubicin, gemcitabine) as well as immunomodulatory agents (BCG, interferon). Standard induction courses (weekly intravesical treatments) may be followed by maintenance treatments assuming favorable response.

Management of Non-urothelial Tumors

Non-urothelial carcinomas account for approximately 10 % of bladder cancers. The distinction between primary non-urothelial malignancy and urothelial carcinoma with divergent histologic differentiation can be difficult, if not impossible, to make by urinary cytology alone. These tumors tend to have a more aggressive phenotype, typically presenting with invasive or locally advanced disease [23]. The histologic diagnosis is made by transurethral resection. Complete resection of all visible tumors, when appropriate, is still recommended in order to distinguish between a pure and mixed histology (which even then, is not always possible depending on the sampling). Due to their rarity, prospective randomized trials comparing treatments are lacking. Consideration should strongly be given to a planned multidisciplinary approach, employing surgery, systemic chemotherapy, and radiation on an individualized basis.

Squamous cell carcinoma is the second most common type of bladder cancer, and is often associated with chronic inflammation from Schistosomal infection, recurrent urinary tract infections, chronic indwelling catheterization, and bladder calculi. Radical cystectomy remains the standard treatment for primary squamous cell carcinoma of the bladder. Radiotherapy with concurrent chemotherapy may be given for unresectable or residual disease.

Primary adenocarcinomas may be associated with bladder exstrophy, urachal anomalies, and chronic inflammation of the bladder. Malignancies from other sites (colorectal, prostatic, breast) must be ruled out. Again, due to the rarity of the disease, comparative trials are lacking and the default standard treatment remains radical cystectomy. For urachal carcinomas, wide local excision of the umbilicus and urachal remnant with cystectomy and pelvic lymphadenectomy is indicated. Unlike urothelial carcinomas that tend to be multifocal due to the field effect nature of the urothelium, primary adenocarcinomas tend to be solitary. As such, partial cystectomy of the dome (for urachal-associated tumors) or those located within a diverticulum may be considered in carefully selected cases.

Micropapillary tumors of the urinary tract are a distinct entity with impact on management, especially in the noninvasive stages. Several studies have shown a lower success rate of intravesical therapy for these tumors and hence the option of early radical cystectomy should be discussed with the patient [23].

Neuroendocrine (NE) tumors of the urinary tract have a propensity for systemic involvement. Both pure NE carcinomas as well as urothelial carcinomas with NE differentiation should be managed with a planned multimodality treatment approach [24]. Neoadjuvant systemic chemotherapy followed by radical cystectomy has demonstrated superior outcomes compared with radical cystectomy alone or with adjuvant postoperative chemotherapy [25]. Combination chemotherapy with definitive radiotherapy (analogous to the management of small cell lung cancer) may also be considered in select cases.

Management of the Unsatisfactory Specimen

"Unsatisfactory" specimens may arise for a number of reasons. The management of this should be left at the discretion of the clinician. Depending on the risk for a significant lesion, a repeat specimen may be obtained, if practical. The reason for the "unsatisfactory" collection should be ascertained so that repeat collections will be more likely to yield diagnostic information.

Management

Although a "SHGUC" cytological diagnosis seems to be strongly associated with a subsequent diagnosis of high-grade urothelial lesions, the available data are limited and do not justify considering such diagnosis similar to a "positive for HGUC" diagnosis from the clinical standpoint at the current time. It is recommended that patients with a "SHGUC" diagnosis be clinically actively investigated in order to rule out the presence of a high-grade urothelial lesion. Repeat cytology evaluation in addition to cystoscopy with biopsy of any visible lesions and/or random biopsies of the urothelial tract to rule out an occult urothelial carcinoma in-situ should be considered. Triggering a nephroureterectomy solely based on a "suspicious" upper tract cytology is not encouraged because it can be associated with significant false negative results.

Conclusions

As the end-users of the urine cytology report, we applaud the herculean efforts of the Working Group of The Paris System in standardizing the criteria and methodology, and bringing uniformity to the diagnostic reporting. This will allow more meaningful comparative study. The evaluation and management described above represent only general recommendations to provide insight for the cytopathologist to understand how a given cytologic diagnosis may impact clinical decision-making. The ultimate care of the patient should be individualized based on all available clinical information. Communication between the clinician and cytopathologist is encouraged in order to optimally utilize this powerful diagnostic tool.

References

1. Xylinas E, Kluth LA, Rieken M, Karakiewicz PI, Lotan Y, Shariat SF. Urine markers for detection and surveillance of bladder cancer. Urol Oncol. 2014;32:222–9.
2. Yafi FA, Brimo F, Steinberg J, Aprikian AG, Tanguay S, Kassouf W. Prospective analysis of sensitivity and specificity of urinary cytology and other urinary biomarkers for bladder cancer. Urol Oncol. 2015;33:66. e25–31.
3. Davis R, Jones JS, Barocas DA, Castle EP, Lang EK, Leveillee RJ, et al. Diagnosis, evaluation and follow-up of asymptomatic microhematuria (AMH) in adults: AUA guideline. J Urol. 2012;188:2473–81.
4. Hall MC, Chang SS, Dalbagni G, Pruthi RS, Seigne JD, Skinner EC, et al. Guideline for the management of nonmuscle invasive bladder cancer (stages Ta, T1, and Tis): 2007 update. J Urol. 2007;178:2314–30.
5. Babjuk M, Burger M, Zigeuner R, Shariat SF, van Rhijn BW, Compérat E, et al. EAU guidelines on non-muscle-invasive urothelial carcinoma of the bladder: update 2013. Eur Urol. 2013;64:639–63.
6. Mitra AP, Alemozaffar M, Harris BN, Schuckman AK, Skinner EC, Daneshmand S. Outcomes after urothelial recurrence in bladder cancer patients undergoing radical cystectomy. Urology. 2014;84:1420–6.
7. Picozzi S, Ricci C, Gaeta M, Ratti D, Macchi A, Casellato S, et al. Upper urinary tract recurrence following radical cystectomy for bladder cancer: a meta-analysis on 13,185 patients. J Urol. 2012;188:2046–54.
8. Clark PE, Stein JP, Groshen SG, Miranda G, Cai J, Lieskovsky G, Skinner DG. The management of urethral transitional cell carcinoma after radical cystectomy for invasive bladder cancer. J Urol. 2004;172:1342–7.
9. Sanderson KM, Cai J, Miranda G, Skinner DG, Stein JP. Upper tract urothelial recurrence following radical cystectomy for transitional cell carcinoma of the bladder: an analysis of 1,069 patients with 10-year followup. J Urol. 2007;177:2088–94.
10. Stein JP, Penson DF, Wu SD, Skinner DG. Pathological guidelines for orthotopic urinary diversion in women with bladder cancer: a review of the literature. J Urol. 2007;178:756–60.
11. Kamat AM, Hegarty PK, Gee JR, Clark PE, Svatek RS, Hegarty N, et al. ICUD-EAU international consultation on bladder cancer 2012: screening, diagnosis, and molecular markers. Eur Urol. 2013;63:4–15.
12. Bubendorf L, Piaton E. UroVysion(R) multiprobe FISH in the triage of equivocal urinary cytology cases. Ann Pathol. 2012;32(6):e52–6. 438–43.
13. Yoder BJ, Skacel M, Hedgepeth R, Babineau DF, Ulchaker JC, Liou LS, et al. Reflex UroVysion testing of bladder cancer surveillance patients with equivocal or negative urine cytology: a prospective study with focus on the natural history of anticipatory positive findings. Am J Clin Pathol. 2007;127:295–301.
14. Skacel M, Fahmy M, Brainard JA, Pettay JD, Biscotti CV, Liou LS. Multitarget fluorescence in situ hybridization assay detects transitional cell carcinoma in the majority of patients with bladder cancer and atypical or negative urine cytology. J Urol. 2003;169:2101–5.
15. Casey RG, Catto JW, Cheng L, Cookson MS, Herr H, Shariat S, et al. Diagnosis and management of urothelial carcinoma in situ of the lower urinary tract: a systematic review. Eur Urol. 2015;67:876–88.
16. Daneshmand S, Schuckman AK, Bochner BH, Cookson MS, Downs TM, Gomella LG, et al. Hexaminolevulinate blue-light cystoscopy in non-muscle-invasive bladder cancer: review of the clinical evidence and consensus statement on appropriate use in the USA. Nat Rev Urol. 2014;11:589–96.

17. Gayed BA, Seideman C, Lotan Y. Cost-effectiveness of fluorescence in situ hybridization in patients with atypical cytology for the detection of urothelial carcinoma. J Urol. 2013;190:1181–6.
18. Herr HW. Randomized trial of narrow-band versus white-light cystoscopy for restaging (second-look) transurethral resection of bladder tumors. Eur Urol. 2015;67:605–8.
19. Lerner SP, Goh A. Novel endoscopic diagnosis for bladder cancer. Cancer. 2015;121: 169–78.
20. Stenzl A, Burger M, Fradet Y, Mynderse LA, Soloway MS, Witjes JA, et al. Hexaminolevulinate guided fluorescence cystoscopy reduces recurrence in patients with nonmuscle invasive bladder cancer. J Urol. 2010;184:1907–13.
21. Witjes JA, Babjuk M, Gontero P, Jacqmin D, Karl A, Kruck S, et al. Clinical and cost effectiveness of hexaminolevulinate-guided blue-light cystoscopy: evidence review and updated expert recommendations. Eur Urol. 2014;66:863–71.
22. Kamat AM, Witjes JA, Brausi M, Soloway M, Lamm D, Persad R, et al. Defining and treating the spectrum of intermediate risk nonmuscle invasive bladder cancer. J Urol. 2014;192:305–15.
23. Willis D, Kamat AM. Nonurothelial bladder cancer and rare variant histologies. Hematol Oncol Clin North Am. 2015;29:237–52.
24. Quek ML, Nichols PW, Yamzon J, Daneshmand S, Miranda G, Cai J, et al. Radical cystectomy for primary neuroendocrine tumors of the bladder: The University of Southern California experience. J Urol. 2005;174:93–6.
25. Siefker-Radtke AO, Dinney CP, Abrahams NA, Moran C, Shen Y, Pisters LL, et al. Evidence supporting preoperative chemotherapy for small cell carcinoma of the bladder: a retrospective review of the M.D. Anderson Cancer experience. J Urol. 2004;172:481–4.

Afterword: The Paris System for Reporting Urinary Cytology

Dorothy L. Rosenthal, Eva M. Wojcik, and Daniel F.I. Kurtycz

The primary goal of The Paris System Working Group was standardizing the terminology for reporting urinary cytology based upon histopathology and clinical outcomes. Soon after the initiation of this project, we realized that much of our knowledge base was anecdotal, poorly defined, inadequately studied, or uninvestigated. Therefore, the Working Group depended not only upon the extant medical literature but also considered the data from newly initiated and completed studies that were needed to reach the goal.

From the initial meeting in Paris, we have agreed that detection of High Grade Urothelial Carcinoma is the ultimate goal of urine cytology. Therefore, the entire system was built based on this principle. As a consequence, one of our goals has been to define the risk of HGUC for each diagnostic category based upon tissue confirmation and clinical outcome. This goal, however, can only be accomplished if the standardized terminology is used for defining risk related to the initial diagnostic categories. As such, prospective studies will have to be done to define those risks.

The decision to emphasize HGUC was based most importantly on clinical significance but also on pathogenetic bases of urothelial carcinoma. Although we have presented these pathways in a very simplistic way, we understand that a significant body of work has yet to be done to confirm that low-grade urothelial neoplasms are not carcinomas. As a remedy for this general ignorance, we decided to divide our knowledge of the pathogenesis of Bladder Cancer into two major categories: those causes of cellular neoplastic changes that have been verified by molecular and genetic tests, and those that are still theories or totally unexplored.

This First Edition of The Paris System for Reporting Urinary Cytology (2015) has covered the morphology of cytologic changes from benign to malignant, and has modestly stated what we believe to be generally accepted causes of these changes. Many of the ancillary tests are still in the investigative phase of their development (see Chap. 9) and are in serious need of large clinical trials to validate their clinical reliability and reproducibility among individuals and laboratories.

D.L. Rosenthal et al. (eds.), *The Paris System for Reporting Urinary Cytology*,
DOI 10.1007/978-3-319-22864-8

In anticipation of The Second Edition, the editors, DR, EW, and DK, have asked the Corresponding Authors of the Working Groups to provide us with a Wish List, i.e., those aspects relative to the topic of their chapter that are in immediate need of investigation. The major purpose of this list, summarized as an appendix to this Afterword, is to stimulate seminal research by medical scientists. We also hope that funding agencies, whether governmental, philanthropic or private industry, will step forward and turn this Grass Roots effort into a major force in combatting Bladder Cancer. As the world's population ages, bladder cancer will become more of a financial burden than it already is, worthy of effective methods of prevention, and early noninvasive detection methods resulting in minimal procedures for effective cures.

Future Clinical and Research Needs for All Diagnostic Categories of The Paris System for Reporting Urinary Cytology

General essentials to assure the longevity of The Paris System

1. Determine the reporting rates of all categories after proper usage of the criteria has occurred for a significant period of time.
2. Perform outcome and interobserver reproducibility studies with the updated criteria.
3. Relate risk for the development of HGUC to the cytologic categories.
4. Establish clear-cut management guidelines based upon outcomes and with input from Urologic Surgeons and acceptance of patients.
5. Consider whether subsequent urothelial tumors are a recurrence of the initial tumor or a new lesion.

Chapter 1: Pathogenesis

1. Conduct further molecular studies to confirm or disprove that hyperplastic and dysplastic pathways are separate in the pathogenesis of urothelial neoplasms.
2. Further evaluate the concept that low grade urothelial neoplasms (LGUNs) are not "carcinomas".

Chapter 2: Specimen Adequacy

1. Define essential variables, e.g., optimal minimum and maximum volume of voided urines, cellularity necessary for diagnosis of HGUC, preservation of cellular integrity dependent upon length of time between collection and processing.
2. Establish when the term "inadequate" is appropriate, and the clinical implications.

Chapter 3: Negative for HGUC (NHGUC)

1. Catalogue outcomes of all entities included within the NHGUC category.
2. Explore whether any of the "benign" entities, especially Polyoma virus and calculi, have a causal relationship with urothelial cancers.

Chapter 4: Atypical Urothelial Cells (AUC)

1. Construct studies to refine criteria and meaningfully reduce the size of the AUC category.
2. Compare use of the category among laboratories of various sizes and risk levels of patients.

Chapter 5: Suspicious for HGUC (SHGUC)

1. Define the cytological categories of "suspicious for HGUC" and "positive for HGUC" in terms of their association with subsequent histological HGUC diagnoses to determine whether they should remain separate categories.
2. Establish management guidelines for a "suspicious" diagnosis based on the results of future large studies.

Chapter 6: HGUC

1. Define the specificity and sensitivity of HGUC cytology for detecting HGUC on biopsy, depending upon the type of cytologic sample obtained.
2. Design large prospective studies to establish risk of recurrence and invasion based upon grade predicted by cytologic diagnosis.

Chapter 7: LGUN

1. Construct studies that are adequately powered to achieve statistical significance in order to establish the clinical utility of the LGUN category.
2. Decide whether any lesions within the LGUN category are truly carcinomas, i.e., capable of invading and metastasizing, and whether these lesions can progress from LGUC to HGUC.

Chapter 8: Non-urothelial

1. Evaluate clinical data from major academic centers to assess the success of morphology and immunohistochemistry for cytological detection of non-urothelial malignancies of the urinary tract.
2. Investigate application of innovative molecular and genetic tests to aid in the identification of sources of non-urothelial cancers of the urinary tract as well as determine the cell of origin in primary non-urothelial tumors.

Chapter 9: Ancillary Tests

1. Prospectively compare the performance of novel tests on the sensitivity and negative predictive value of AUC and SHGUC categories.
2. Determine whether surveillance guidelines can be changed using currently approved ancillary tests (e.g., U-FISH and uCyt) for patients with urothelial carcinoma depending on individual risk factors.
3. Establish the cost-effectiveness of ancillary testing across different countries and health care systems.

Chapter 10: Preparation

1. Determine whether time, temperature, and chemical composition of urine impact collection and processing.
2. Establish evidence-based recommendations for collecting urine specimens (e.g., voided early a.m. vs. discard-hydrate-void; voided vs. catheterized vs. washing).

Chapter 11: Clinical Management

1. Explore new technologies to improve the accuracy of cystoscopy, such as fluorescence-assisted cystoscopy, narrow band imaging, among others, that have been introduced or will be coming down the pipeline.
2. Perform prospective clinical trials to see how these tests can be integrated with cytology to enhance its performance.

Index

D.L. Rosenthal et al. (eds.), *The Paris System for Reporting Urinary Cytology*,
DOI 10.1007/978-3-319-22864-8

Printed by Printforce, the Netherlands